PRAISE FOR THE FIRST EDITION OF

— GENETICALLY ENGINEERED FOOD —

"It is great that Ronnie Cummins and Ben Lilliston have had the courage and the dedication to research the controversial subject of genetically engineered foods so thoroughly. Every aspect is covered—health hazards, effects on the environment, where to shop, what to avoid—allowing us to choose where our interests lie and, from this, check resources and make educated decisions. This guide must surely become the bible for the concerned consumer."

—NORA POUILLON, chef/owner of Restaurant Nora, Washington, D.C., the country's first certified organic restaurant, and Asia Nora

"Consumers have known intuitively that they don't want to eat genetically engineered foods. Now they know why. Ronnie Cummins and Ben Lilliston persuasively outline the case against this mass experiment on our food, and give the public useful tools for ways to avoid genetic contamination when they buy food. Anyone who eats should read *Genetically Engineered Food*. It is indispensable as a basic primer, a resource guide, and a call to action."

—CHARLES MARGULIS, Greenpeace genetic engineering specialist

"Cummins and Lilliston are clear, accurate, and compelling. If you want to understand the dangers of genetically engineered food, this is the book you need. And if you want to make safe food choices for your family, this is the book you should buy."

—CHERYL LONG, senior editor of *Organic Gardening* magazine

"I breathed a sigh of relief as I picked up this book. Finally, there's a reliable source of information for consumers on the confusing subject of genetically engineered foods. In clear language, Cummins and

Lilliston guide us to greater knowledge...and greater hopefulness. If you only read one book on GE foods, this should be the one."

—PEGGY O'MARA, editor and publisher, *Mothering* Magazine

"Cummins and Lilliston are top investigative writers and activists who spill the beans about what's wrong with genetically engineered food and how to avoid them. Everyone who eats needs this book."

—JOHN STAUBER, coauthor of *Toxic Sludge is Good For You* and *Mad Cow USA*

"A fundamental right of consumers is knowing what kind of foods they are purchasing. Genetically engineered foods are taking this right away from consumers. This book helps make the marketplace more democratic, giving consumers the information they need to make choices in buying food for their families. I look forward to seeing this book on every coffee table in America."

—RENSKE VAN STAVEREN, national coordinator, Genetic Engineering Action Network, USA

"Cummins and Lilliston's self-defense guide is a boon. Their comprehensive reporting on GE food explains the risks and the politics of all this sci-fi farming, along with shopping strategies to help you avoid buying, say, a gene-spliced Twinkie."

—*Isthmus*

"Thick with information about finding healthful food and fighting for a sustainable, humane, and equitable food and agriculture system, this book ably outlines the ideas and the values that ought to frame any discussion of food policy."

—*Capitol Times*

GENETICALLY ENGINEERED FOOD

A Self-Defense Guide for Consumers

RONNIE CUMMINS AND BEN LILLISTON
FOREWORD BY FRANCES MOORE LAPPÉ

MARLOWE & COMPANY
NEW YORK

GENETICALLY ENGINEERED FOOD:
A Self-Defense Guide for Consumers

Copyright © 2000, 2004 Ronnie Cummins and Ben Lilliston
Foreword © 2004 Frances Moore Lappé

Published by
Marlowe & Company
An Imprint of Avalon Publishing Group Incorporated
245 West 17th Street • 11th Floor
New York, NY 10011

Library of Congress Cataloging-in-Publication Data
Cummins, Ronnie
Genetically engineered food: a self-defense guide for consumers/Ronnie
Cummins and Ben Lilliston; foreword by Andrew Kimbrell.—[2nd , rev. ed.]
p. cm.
Includes bibliographical references
ISBN 1-56924-469-3
1. Food—Biotechnology—Popular works. 2. Crops—Genetic engineering—
Popular works.
I. Lilliston, Ben. II. Title.

TP248.65.F66C85 2004
363.19'2—dc22   2004045565

ISBN 1-56924-469-3

9   8   7   6   5   4   3   2   1

Designed by Pauline Neuwirth, Neuwirth & Associates, Inc.

Printed in the United States of America
Distributed by Publishers Group West

DEDICATION

FOR THE consumers and farmers worldwide who are helping to move us toward a food and agricultural system, which is organic, sustainable, humane, and equitable.

CONTENTS

FOREWORD
by Frances Moore Lappé

CONGRATULATIONS. If you've picked up this book, you're a fortunate person indeed. You're in for an awakening; a rude one to be sure, but a jolt that will change the way you see your world. And, I believe, it can also change the way you see your own power.

Here Ronnie Cummins and Ben Lilliston, two dogged researchers and courageous truth-tellers, inform us that we Americans have been enlisted in the biggest nutritional experiment ever conducted on humans—on any species for that matter. Ethicists hold that experiments on humans require our informed consent. However, those carrying out this particular experiment, the introduction of genetically engineered food (and especially seeds, where it all starts), not only failed to ask for our consent; they even failed to tell us the experiment was underway.

Just since 1996, genetically engineered seeds have spread 40 fold to cover 167 million acres around the world—two-thirds of those acres are right here in the U.S. So we Americans are truly the world's guinea pigs. The reason is not merely that the primary developer of genetically modified seeds, Monsanto—which controls over 90 percent of the market—is based in this country. There is a deeper factor that can alert us to a crisis within our democracy itself.

In many other countries, governments and citizens have actively, vociferously, and publicly debated whether spreading an untested technology—one capable of altering ecological systems and human health—is a good idea. Most have said, "No, given the high stakes, we must be cautious." And where genetically modified products have been allowed on the market, governments have typically insisted they be clearly labeled. (Even China, hardly a paragon of concern for its citizens' welfare, requires labeling of genetically engineered food!)

But not here in the U.S. Before there was any public awareness, much less debate, our government—at the urging of corporate developers of genetic engineering—declared that genetically modified foods are no different from those conventionally produced. Rigorous testing and oversight, it was said, are simply unnecessary. Government scientists who raised questions were rebuked and pushed out. Even today, despite petitions from hundreds of thousands of Americans, there is no labeling of products containing genetically engineered ingredients. Sadly, while as many as two-thirds of the items in a typical supermarket contain them, most Americans believe they've never eaten a genetically modified food.

Thus while Cummins and Lilliston appropriately call this highly useful book a "self-defense guide for consumers," to me it is also a wake-up call for citizens. For I have come to see the rapid spread of genetically engineered seeds as a symptom of our silencing, the silencing of a people that results from the usurpation by unelected powers—corporations—of our democratic rights to protect ourselves and shape our own future. Many of our nation's founders understood well that democracy has an economic foundation—that, as Justice Louis Brandeis (1846–1941) said much later, "We can have democracy in this country, or we can have great wealth concentrated in the hands of a few, but we can't have both."

Fortunately, an awakening to this assault on democracy is spurring a movement of citizens on every continent. Recently, for example, residents of Mendocino County, California, made history by banning the planting of genetically engineered seeds (despite the fact that corporate opponents outspent the people's campaign by almost 7 to 1). By reading this book and then making real, informed choices, you will take part in this historic possibility.

Frances Moore Lappé
Cambridge, Massachusetts
April 6, 2004

FRANCES MOORE LAPPÉ is a renowned food activist and the author of numerous books, including the 3-million-copy bestseller *Diet for a Small Planet*, and coauthor of *Hope's Edge*. She is the cofounder of The Small Planet Fund and Food First. She lives in Cambridge, Massachusetts

PREFACE

FOUR YEARS after the first edition of this book, the controversy over genetically engineered (GE) foods and crops continues to escalate. New scientific evidence on environmental and human health hazards fuels the debate, as does the food industry's stubborn refusal, at least in the United States and Canada, to label GE foods. Meanwhile requirements for labeling and traceability have all but driven GE foods off the market in Europe. Major European food companies have begun requiring that GE soybeans, corn, and cotton seeds be removed from animal feeds as well as consumer products. In response the United States has filed a formal trade complaint against the EU at the World Trade Organization, although almost no one expects Europeans to accept "Frankenfoods," as the EU press has dubbed them, no matter what the WTO rules. Wall Street remains skeptical about the future of gene-spliced crops. Monsanto, whose patented seeds account for 91 percent of all GE field crops, has suffered recently from a sharp decline in profits. Farmers and rural communities are still voicing misgivings about the supposed benefits of transgenic crops, with lawsuits by Monsanto against farmers, and counter-lawsuits by farmers against Monsanto and other biotech firms increasing.

Ten years after the introduction of agricultural biotechnology, only four GE crops are being grown on a commercial scale: soy-beans, corn, cotton, and canola—with most of these crops being funneled into animal feed. Among these genetically modified crops only two agricultural traits have been added—herbicide resistance (75 percent of all GE crops), pesticide resistance (17 percent), or both (8 percent). And these four GE crops are still only being grown, for all practical purposes, in four nations: the United States, Canada, Argentina, and China. In perhaps the most frightening recent development, an unapproved genetically engineered biopharm crop designed to produce a vaccine contam-inated 500,000 bushels of soybeans. Despite clear dangers, the biotech industry is promoting biopharm crops as the next wave of this radical technology. And of course the most important factor in the biotech debate is that ordinary consumers and parents are still raising questions, educating themselves, and taking action.

As we pointed out four years ago, what once appeared to be the inevitable dawn of the Biotech Century for American agriculture may well turn out to be the beginning of a serious and thoughtful reexamination of how food is produced. As part of this reexamina-tion, we are already seeing phenomenal expansion in the demand for organic foods in the United States, Canada, Europe, Japan, and other nations. In 2003 farmers in 110 nations produced and sold $25 billion in certified organic crops and foods, while global sales of GMOs (genetically modified organisms) leveled off at approximately $4.25 billion.

The debate over genetically engineered foods and crops, includ-ing GE animal drugs such as Monsanto's Bovine Hormone (rBGH) and food crops laced with pharmaceutical drugs and industrial chemicals, may last for decades. However, as Europe has shown, the ultimate arbiter of power in this debate is the consumer. Marketplace pressure can change the landscape quickly. If U.S. consumers continue to take action in their everyday lives—following the food-buying and food-preparation suggestions in the second half of this book—genetically engineered foods will be short-lived. Food companies, restaurants, supermarkets, institutional investors—even politicians—recognize what affects their bottom line. If American consumers reject genetically engineered foods, putting their food dollars where their concerns and values lie, this technology will fail.

We are happy that the first edition of this book has sold so well as to warrant a second, updated edition. This is but one indication that public concern and awareness is growing about this radical new technology. Please read this book and pass it around to your friends, but also be prepared to take action for the future of our food. The old adage, you are what you eat, has never been more applicable. Bon Appetit!

WHAT'S FOR DINNER?
The Genetically Engineered Foods Controversy

WALK THROUGH the aisles of any supermarket in America. Sit down to eat in just about any restaurant, school cafeteria, workplace lunchroom, hospital, or airplane. Open your cupboards and refrigerator. Look at what's cooking in your oven, microwave, or frying pan, or what's on your fork, your spoon, in your cup or drinking glass. . . . You can't see, smell, taste, or feel the difference. And you can't read about it on food labels or restaurant menus (at least in the United States). But you and your family are now part of a vast culinary and biological experiment—dining on an expanding menu of genetically engineered foods. Foods unlike any foods consumed in human history.

Genetically engineered foods (see the box below for other comparable, frequently used terms) have been big news in Europe, Asia, and Australia for the last several years. European and

Japanese consumers have led the way, resoundingly rejecting American gene-food exports and forcing major supermarket chains and food manufacturers overseas to remove genetically engineered foods and ingredients from the marketplace. Now individual consumers, consumer advocates, research scientists, environmental organizations, farmers, and other concerned citizens in the United States and Canada are joining the debate—helping to raise substantive questions about the risks—potential and known—of this new and highly touted technology. The most urgent question being asked by more and more people worldwide is: Are genetically engineered foods harmful to human health and the environment?

DIFFERENT NAMES, SAME MEANING

Around the world, and even in this book, you will find a number of different terms or abbreviations for genetically engineered (GE) foods and organisms. Many of these terms mean the same thing, but reflect different cultural biases relative to language. Below is a short list of common terms and definitions.

- Genetically engineered (GE)—This is the standard U.S. term for a process in which foreign genes are spliced into a non-related species, creating an entirely new organism.
- Genetically modified (GM)—The same as GE, this term is more widely used in Europe because it translates more easily among different languages.
- Genetically modified organism (GMO)—The actual organism that is created through genetic engineering.
- Biotech foods, gene-foods, bioengineered foods, gene-altered foods, transgenic foods—Foods that have been created through genetic engineering.
- Frankenfoods—Another term for the above, refering to the story of Frankenstein and science gone bad.
- Biopharm—GE crops designed to produce pharmaceutical drugs and industrial chemicals.

Not since the nuclear power debates in the late 1970s has there been such controversy over a new technology of this magnitude. Like their counterparts in the nuclear industry forty years ago, the proponents of agricultural genetic engineering offer consumers a cornucopia of benefits, promising to end world hunger, improve public health, and reduce pesticide use. They confidently proclaim that gene-foods are safe. They cite industry-sponsored studies and invoke the names of national and international regulatory agencies that have given several dozen varieties of genetically engineered crops and foods clearance for commercialization. But like their predecessors in the nuclear industry a generation ago, the more they talk, and the more independent scientific evidence accumulates, the less credible proponents of agricultural genetic engineering seem. What's becoming clear is that:

- Agricultural genetic engineering is a radical and unpredictable new technology.
- GE foods are not being adequately safety-tested for possible damage to our health.
- GE crops are not being adequately safety-tested for possible damage to the environment
- GE crops overall do not require fewer pesticides than conventional crops, and in most cases require more.
- GE foods are no more nutritious than conventional foods.
- GE crops are not addressing global hunger through higher yields.
- Genetically engineered ingredients are pervasive in processed foods in the U.S. and Canada, and yet they are not labeled.
- Agricultural genetic engineering has negative social and economic impacts on family farmers and rural communities in the U.S. and around the world.
- Mounting scientific evidence indicates that genetically engineered foods and crops may present serious hazards for our health and our environment.

- Once released onto the market and into the environment, genetically engineered material cannot be contained.

A GROWING CONCERN IN NORTH AMERICA

ALTHOUGH THE volume of the genetically engineered foods debate is not yet as intense in North America as it is in Europe, Japan, Australia, and a number of other nations, the tenor of the discussion is steadily—and now very quickly—rising in the United States. In fact, it is clear that Americans are increasingly nervous about this new and controversial technology, and strongly feel the need for additional information. Public concern in the U.S. over gene-foods is not new, however. As far back as 1994, when the first two genetically engineered foods were introduced in the United States, there were clear signs of consumer skepticism. The introduction of the Bovine Growth Hormone, injected into dairy cows to force them to produce more milk, led to the tripling of the market for organic milk. The Flavr Savr tomato, which had been gene-altered for longer shelf life, fell flat on its face when consumers refused to buy it. (We will discuss these and other gene-foods in greater depth later in the book.)

National polls repeatedly reflect the depth of concern among Americans about genetically engineered food. An ABC News poll in June 2001 found 93 percent of U.S. consumers want labels on GE foods, while a Rutgers University poll in November 2001 found 90 percent supporting labeling. Another ABC News poll released in July 2003 found that 92 percent of Americans wanted labels, while 62 percent of women said they would prefer to avoid purchasing GE food for their families. Again and again, polls of consumers over the past decade find that 80–95 percent of Americans want genetically engineered foods to be labeled—primarily so that we can avoid buying or consuming them.[1]

AMERICA'S ALTERED HARVEST: STARTLING STATISTICS ON KEY CROPS

WHILE MANY consumers have remained anxious or concerned about genetically engineered foods, a significant percentage of farmers in the U.S. have embraced the new technology. By 2003, over 101 million acres of GE crops were planted in the U.S., representing almost 10 percent of the total acreage of our nation's farmland and pasture. The American gene-altered harvest of 2003 included approximately:

- 81 percent of U.S. soybeans
- 40 percent of U.S. corn
- 73 percent of U.S. cotton
- Over 50 percent of the U.S. and Canadian canola crop

Source: U.S. Department of Agriculture

In addition to these genetically engineered crops, an estimated two million of the U.S.'s nine million dairy cows are being injected regularly with recombinant Bovine Growth Hormone (sometimes referred to as rBGH or rBST). Recombinant Bovine Growth Hormone is banned in Europe, Canada, Japan, and every other industrialized nation except the United States, Brazil, and Mexico.

Since 1991, biotechnology companies have conducted over 300 field trials of so-called biopharm crops in the U.S. It is probable that contamination of the U.S. food supply with genetically engineered pharmaceuticals has already occurred—we have no way of knowing due to the extreme degree of secrecy surrounding the locations of biopharm field trials and the nature of the drugs and chemicals they are engineered to produce.

By the beginning of 2004, a full menu of GE foods, crops, and microorganisms have made their way into kitchens and shopping carts nationwide. Analysts estimate that a full 60–75 percent of processed foods commonly found on supermarket shelves or at your favorite restaurant would "test positive" for the presence of gene-altered soy, corn, cottonseed, canola, and ingredients derived from these genetically engineered crops.

GENE-FOODS ARE EVERYWHERE—
IN MANY OF THE FOODS THAT WE EAT!

ALTHOUGH GENETICALLY engineered foods are neither required to be safety-tested nor to be labeled, they are now part of your everyday diet.[2] According to laboratory tests carried out on behalf of the *New York Times* and *Consumer Reports*, as well as disclosures by food and biotechnology companies, your daily intake of genetically modified organisms (GMOs) may now come from the following foods, among others:

- baby foods
- baking mixes
- breakfast cereals
- cooking oils
- corn
- corn chips
- corn sweeteners
- dairy products
- infant formula
- margarine
- papayas
- popcorn
- radicchio
- salad dressings
- soy burgers
- squash

Scores of other genetically engineered foods and ingredients are poised for commercialization—that is, for sale to consumers, farmers (in seed form), and food manufacturers. Wherever foods are sold or served, it is becoming increasingly difficult for you to avoid purchasing or ingesting genetically engineered foods—without your knowledge.

How did this ever-expanding menu of GE foods get into our shopping carts, kitchens, restaurants, and nursing homes, and onto our kids' school lunch trays? How did we get into a situation where much, if not most, of the food we eat every day contains GMOs, without our approval or consent and without—at least until very recently—even our knowledge? And why have we as citizens been largely excluded from the discussions and policy decisions on genetically engineered foods?

GROWING DOUBTS, MORE QUESTIONS FOR CONSUMERS

AS GE crops become more prevalent, they are subjected to greater scrutiny. Unfortunately, upon closer examination the technology raises doubts rather than confidence. A number of events over the past five years have catalyzed public debate among the media and public:

- In 1998, the prestigious British Medical Association (the equivalent of the American Medical Association, or AMA, in the U.S.) called for a moratorium on all genetically engineered foods because they may not be safe;
- In the 1990s, after reviewing the scientific data, Canada, the European Union, Japan, and a number of other industrialized nations banned Bovine Growth Hormone;
- In the fall of 2000, an illegal, possibly allergenic variety of genetically engineered corn, called StarLink, got into the U.S. food supply, prompting a massive recall of over 300 brand-name products. Three years later StarLink was still showing up in trace amounts in U.S. corn exports.
- In 2002, the U.S. government admitted that two field plots of transgenic corn in Iowa and Nebraska, gene-spliced with

experimental pharmaceutical drugs, had contaminated millions of pounds of feed corn and soybeans. Following the incident, major food corporations such as General Mills and Frito-Lay warned the government to ban the planting of GE "pharm" crops in which industrial chemicals and pharaceutical drugs are gene-spliced into food crops such as corn.

Likewise, more Americans are asking why our government agencies designated to protect us—the Food and Drug Administration, the U.S. Department of Agriculture, and the Environmental Protection Agency—have not been more active in regulating genetically engineered foods.

NO LABELS ON GENE-FOODS: DENYING YOUR RIGHT TO KNOW

THERE IS one fundamental reason why gene-foods are now being grown, sold, and served all over the U.S.: because the corporations that have invested billions of dollars in this new technology have successfully lobbied U.S. government agencies to allow genetically engineered foods to enter our food chain and the environment virtually undetected. In a span of only ten years, the agricultural biotechnology industry has not only managed to begin to transform many of the foods you eat everyday, but, even more amazingly, have managed to do so, for the most part, without your knowledge.

Imagine a pharmaceutical company slipping an entirely different chemical or additive into a well-known over-the-counter drug, and continuing to market the drug as the same well-known drug—never telling the consumer about the different chemical composition. Remarkably, this is what the agriculture biotech industry is doing to our food—they are changing its makeup and selling it to us as if it's the same food we've eaten all our lives.

The biotech industry's opposition to labeling is not surprising.

As Norman Braksick, the president of Asgrow Seed Co., a biotechnology seed company (now owned by Monsanto) admitted to the *Kansas City Star* as far back as 1994, "If you put a label on a genetically engineered food you might as well put a skull and crossbones on it."[3]

Unfortunately, many of the current biotech companies do not have a good track record when it comes to informing the public about potential hazards of their products. Many of today's largest agricultural biotechnology companies (some refer to themselves as "Life Science" companies) are the corporations (or their successors) that in the last half of the twentieth century introduced toxic pesticides, DDT, Agent Orange, PCBs, dioxin, and many other pollutants and carcinogens. As far back as 1962, Rachel Carson warned in her then-groundbreaking book, *Silent Spring*, that putting chemical companies in charge of our food chain was not a good idea.

THE QUESTIONS WE SHOULD ALL BE ASKING

BECAUSE GENETIC engineering is so startlingly different than anything we've ever encountered, it raises a number of important questions—many of which have yet to be answered. What exactly is genetic engineering, and how dangerous is this new technology? How does genetic engineering differ from traditional plant breeding and animal husbandry? Is gene-splicing an exact science, or is it more like William Tell shooting an apple off your head wearing a blindfold (to paraphrase Dr. Arpad Pusztai, a prominent biochemist in Great Britain)? What are the primary human health, environmental, social, and ethical hazards of genetic engineering?

What about reports that gene-foods may contain:

- harmful allergens
- toxins or poisons

- antibiotic-resistant genes
- infective viral agents
- lowered nutritional values
- greater pesticide residues
- substances causing human immune system damage
- substances that increase cancer hazards

What about reports of GE crops:

- killing Monarch butterflies
- killing beneficial insects
- damaging soil fertility
- damaging animal health
- creating "superweeds"
- creating "superpests"
- creating new virulent plant viruses
- causing genetic pollution and genetic drift
- contaminating conventional and organic crops
- threatening wildlife, and biodiversity
- giving rise to harmful plant pathogens, such as the fusarium fungus

What about the negative impact of genetic engineering on family farmers and rural communities in the U.S., as well as subsistence farmers and rural villagers around the world? What about contracts farmers must sign that prohibit them from saving and replanting their own seeds and allow seed companies to inspect their property at any time? Are GE crops really improving yields? What about the claims of the agricultural biotechnology industry that GE crops will feed the hungry, promote sustainable agriculture, and enhance public health?

And are U.S. government regulatory agencies doing all they can to protect public health and the environment? Can food corporations in the U.S. be pressured to reject genetic engineering as they have in Europe and Japan?

WHAT WILL THIS BOOK DO FOR YOU?
WHAT CAN YOU DO FOR YOURSELF
AND YOUR FAMILY?

GENETICALLY ENGINEERED Food: A Self-Defense Guide for Consumers has two primary objectives. Our first goal is to help you to clearly understand why you should be concerned about purchasing or consuming genetically engineered foods in terms of human health hazards. We'll also alert you to the risks that genetically engineered crops are posing to the environment, and help you to understand why a genetically engineered future is not one we want our children, our children's children, or any future generations to inherit. Our second goal is to provide you with the practical steps and strategies you can take to defend yourself and your family from the hazards and uncertainties of foods derived from genetically modified organisms. The good news is that there is a lot you *can* do—every day—as you buy groceries, prepare meals, and dine out in restaurants. We will help you to understand what you can tell from reading ingredients labels on food packages, and what you should be concerned about when you go out to a restaurant, or when your kids eat lunch at school. We will give you more ideas than you may have ever thought possible for finding GE-free and organic foods in your local area. We will also provide you with the names of nationwide and regional supermarket chains that have publicly stated policies about selling GMO foods, and we'll tell you where to turn if you want to find out the policy of your local grocery store. Finally, we will arm you with the brand names of hundreds of organic foods and of certain "natural" foods labeled as GE-free, and we'll tell you which conventional foods are GE-free.

Many of the strategies we present and our suggestions for where and how to shop and what to buy may be new to you. You may find yourself asking: Can I really shop for food any other way than I do now? But the fact is, changing your food-buying habits is not as difficult as it might at first seem, especially as the number of outlets selling organic and GE-free foods continues to increase nationwide.

We believe that the more you understand about the technology behind the genetic engineering of food organisms, the more alarmed you will become. This book is **a self-defense guide** for you and other consumers, and it is a call for you to take action—in your kitchen, in your local grocery stores or at your local farmer's market, at your favorite restaurants and your children's schools, or in the offices of your local, state, and federal representatives.

There are few things in life more fundamental than food. It is no exaggeration to say that we as individuals and we as a society are what we eat. Armed with the proper information and determination, you can regain your fundamental right to know what is in your food. You, along with your family and neighbors, can reassert your free choice and sovereignty—both in your own kitchens, in the public marketplace, and in the body politic. The controversy over genetically engineered foods represents a turning point for our society. We all have the power to make a choice: to choose between harmful, unsustainable agriculture or sustainable farming, to choose between genetically engineered food and safe food. These choices lie within our hands, within reach of our wallets, our forks and our knives. We hope that this book helps you to decide the nature of the food you eat—and helps you to make a GE-free future a reality.

SNAPSHOTS FROM THE GLOBAL FOOD FIGHT OVER GE FOODS 1994–2004

A dozen chefs in white hats, flanked by a bank of TV cameras and news photographers, dump cartons of milk on the sidewalk in front of an upscale supermarket in New York City, protesting U.S. government approval of the world's first genetically engineered food product, recombinant Bovine Growth Hormone. A lively contingent of demonstrators, carrying banners and signs, burst into Monsanto's headquarters in London and occupy the executive offices. Masked eco-guerrillas, under the cover of darkness, uproot an experimental plot of genetically engineered corn in Germany. Activists in a rubber dinghy block a grain ship from unloading its cargo of GE soybeans in Antwerp, Belgium. A Greenpeace truck, sporting a banner "Tony, Don't Swallow Bill's Seed," dumps five tons of gene-altered soybeans on the sidewalk in front of British Prime Minister Tony Blair's residence in London. Sierra Club and Council of Canadians activists leaflet consumers coming in and out of a supermarket in Toronto. Consumer representatives bow and present petitions with the signatures of two million citizens to Japanese government officials in Tokyo—demanding mandatory labeling of genetically engineered foods. . . .

Heated debate breaks out on the floor of the European Parliament in Strasbourg, France, as the Green Party delegation calls for a complete moratorium on GE foods. A group of Indian farmers, in Gandhi-style white traditional clothing, stand at the edge of a field and watch as flames engulf a crop of genetically engineered cotton. In front of the international press corps at the World Food Summit in Rome, a half-dozen young women, with anti-GE slogans painted on their bodies, strip naked and disrupt a speech being delivered by Dan Glickman, then-Secretary of the U.S. Department of Agriculture. Protesters climb to the top of the Independence Monument in Mexico City and hang a banner demanding an end to imports of genetically engineered corn from the United States. Farmers in the province of Rio Grande do Sul, Brazil, march in the streets chanting for a ban on imports of GE soybeans. Several hundred protesters, carrying banners and signs, led by a contingent of of young children in Monarch butterfly costumes, picket outside a FDA hearing on GE foods in Chicago. At the "Battle of Seattle" French and American farmers hold a press conference outside a McDonald's restaurant, demanding a ban on genetically engineered foods and the abolition of the World Trade Organization. . . .

Consumer advocates stand outside a Safeway supermarket in San Francisco, holding aloft a box of brand-name taco shells, one of 300 consumer items recalled by the FDA for possibly containing an illegal, likely allergenic variety of GE corn called StarLink. Organic farmers and their lawyers at a press conference in Saskatchewan, Canada, announce a lawsuit against Monsanto and

Aventis for polluting their conola crops with GE crop pollen drift. Several thousand protesters, surrounded by an equal number of heavily armed riot police, march down the street in Sacramento, California, outside an international agricultural summit sponsored by the USDA, designed to promote genetically engineered foods and crops. . . .

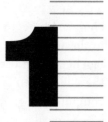

WHAT IS GENETIC ENGINEERING?

THE BUSINESS of genetic engineering is the practice of altering or disrupting the genetic blueprints of living organisms—including plants, animals, microorganisms, and humans—then patenting these altered genes and selling the resulting gene-foods, seeds, or other products for profit. Specifically, laboratory scientists use gene guns, chemical switches called promoters, and bacterial vectors to facilitate the transfer of genetic material between the cells of species that would never be able to breed or propagate in any natural environment. In other words, scientists transfer an indeterminate amount of genetic information or DNA from one or more organisms across species boundaries into another host organism, to create an entirely new genetically engineered organism.

All living organisms, whether bacteria, plants, animals, or human beings, contain DNA—the building blocks of life. DNA is a genetic matrix of chemical proteins stored in the chromosomes within the nucleus of every cell. This genetic matrix is organized into a long, orderly sequence, in the shape of a double helix—imagine a twisted ladder or a spiral staircase—which contains the chemical blueprints and instructions for what cells are supposed to do, which is to manufacture proteins and carry out the basic biochemical processes of birth, life, and death. The DNA inside the cell nucleus is basically the software of life, operating like a computer program to inscribe the instructions for the everyday biochemical activities of the organism.

The technology applied to genetically modify organisms began with research in the early 1970s. At that time molecular biologists started to develop what is called recombinant DNA technology. This new technology is a process that involves transplanting genetic material across species barriers. For the first time, scientists used chemical scissors or enzymes to take genes from bacteria, viruses, and other living organisms and forcibly insert these "foreign" genes into plants, animals, or even humans—and vice versa.

Some forms of recombinant DNA technology, such as using bacteria to copy or make more of a substance such as human insulin, are fairly simple and straightforward. Other forms of genetic engineering, such as splicing an entire package or "cassette" of foreign proteins, viruses, and bacteria into food crops, are more complicated and unpredictable.

Genetic engineers carry out these transplants or gene-splicing operations hoping to transfer a "desirable characteristic" associated with a particular gene in the "donor" organism into a new "host" organism, which will, in turn, exhibit or express this new "desired characteristic." For instance, a common genetically engineered corn was designed to carry a toxic pesticide in every cell to ward off a particularly nasty pest—the corn borer. This new species will then pass on its acquired traits, through heredity, to its offspring.

GENETIC ENGINEERING IS A
REVOLUTIONARY NEW TECHNOLOGY

GENETIC ENGINEERING, although thirty years old, is a revolutionary new technology still in the early experimental stages of development. It enables molecular biologists to permanently alter the essential characteristics or genetic codes of living organisms. This technology has the awesome power to break down fundamental genetic barriers—not only between species but between humans, animals, and plants. Gene engineers all over the world are now snipping, inserting, recombining, rearranging, editing, and programming genetic material. Animal genes and even human genes are being randomly inserted into the chromosomes of plants, fish, and animals, creating heretofore unimaginable transgenic life forms.

"This is probably one of the most technologically powerful developments the world has ever seen," EPA toxicologist Suzanne Wuerthele told four hundred Nebraska farm leaders in March 2000. "It's the biological equivalent of splitting the atom."[1]

For the first time in history, the scientists and corporations using this technology have become, in effect, the architects, builders, and "owners" of life. Life science corporations today not only have patents giving them legal ownership over the process of genetically manipulating living organisms such as soybean plants, but also legal ownership over the newly created organism itself. Thus a farmer does not own the genetically engineered seeds he buys—instead he is leasing the technology from the corporation that holds the patent (more on this in chapter 4).

THE DOWNSIDE OF GENE-SPLICING

THE PROCESS of genetic engineering may sound nifty at first. Over the past two decades, many people have become enthusiastic about this new technology, and have begun to think about the possibilities of literally re-engineering life. Unfortunately, however (as we will discuss in more detail later), living organisms are not designed like machines, with interchangeable parts. Individual genes do not have a one-to-one correspondence with certain "desired characteristics" or traits, and the "surgery" employed in gene-splicing is messy, imprecise, and unpredictable. Instead of producing "superior" breeds of plants, animals, or humans—a sort of a genetic "master race"—a large percentage of genetic transplants end in failure. In fact, only one in thousands of attempts achieves the desired results without undesirable side effects.[2]

All too often, researchers end up with transgenic stillborns, mutants, freaks, and failures, with genetically modified organisms that don't behave like they're supposed to. These genetically modified organisms can act on their internal and external cellular and biological environments in unpredictable and unexpected ways.

One of the first early genetic engineering experiments illustrates the perils of attempting to transfer genetic characteristics from one species to another. In the 1980s, U.S. Department of Agriculture scientists transplanted human genes—genes supposedly associated with human growth—into pigs. By doing so they hoped to make the pigs grow faster, and increase their profitability for farmers. Unfortunately, the outcome of these experiments was not what USDA scientists expected. In one infamous incident, instead of the "superpig" they hoped for, the pig that resulted from this gene experiment developed into a deformed creature, one that was "excessively hairy, lethargic, riddled with arthritis, apparently impotent, and slightly cross-eyed." As if that weren't bad enough, "the pig could barely stand up," according to reports.[3]

The sobering fact is that living organisms—even the simpler ones—in their internal cellular workings and their interrelationships with their surrounding biological ecosystems are infinitely more complex than what humans, with our current levels of understanding, can comprehend, much less successfully "create" or engineer.

GENETIC ENGINEERS know how to remove the DNA of a donor organism, and they have learned how to break through species barriers by shooting pellets of this DNA through biological cell walls into a "host organism." To do so, they have developed "gene guns" or bacterial vectors that can penetrate the cell walls of target organisms and deliver a payload of altered genetic material. *Agribacterium tumefaciens* is one such plant bacteria that scientists use as a vector or a sort of cellular taxi.

While scientists have been able to isolate specific characteristics or traits that they want to insert into a new species, they cannot yet precisely control the location where that trait will be inserted. In other words, they are firing the gene gun or launching the bacterial vector with little idea where the payload of desired traits will crash through the cell walls of the host organism and begin to disrupt its complex biochemical matrix. This random, shotgun-like insertion inevitably causes a disruption of the order and balance of the genes on the host chromosome and can readily result in random and unexpected changes in the biochemical functioning of the cells.

For example, scientists at the University of Chicago looking at genetically engineered plants from the mustard family found that two genetically engineered lines (created using the same process) were significantly different in their ability to crossbreed with plant relatives—attributed to the different location of where the genes were inserted.[4] In another experiment, scientists working to genetically engineer yeast accidentally disrupted its metabolism, resulting in a 40- to 200-fold increase in methyglyoxal (MG)—a toxic substance. This study points to a potential unexpected, and hazardous, effect of genetic engineering, but also the dramatic differences (between 40 and 200 fold) that the location of gene insertion can create.[5]

THE POTENTIAL for unexpected disruptions resulting from the random insertion of DNA from one organism into another are not the only possible perils of genetic engineering. When scientists send the cellular taxi crashing through the cell walls of the host organism, the taxi usually includes a "genetic cassette" or package of altered genes. These cassettes often include several genetic components, including the Cauliflower Mosaic Virus (CaMV), a commonly used viral promoter, which acts as a chemical switch to turn on certain biochemical processes in the cell. Genes in plants have their own promoters, so the genetic engineer brings in the CaMV—an extremely powerful promoter—to overwhelm the gene's own promoter system. The arrival of this genetic cassette in the host organism sets in motion and amplifies a whole series of biochemical reactions.

Unfortunately, the CaVM is such a strong promoter that it can accidentally turn genes on or off, up and down a given chromosome or even in another chromosome.[6] Additionally, there is no way to turn off these chemical switches once they're turned on, and there is no precise way to control the volume or intensity of the specific genes or chemical processes that have been turned on.

The remarkable changes posed by genetic engineering on the normal functions of a plant sometimes result in something called "gene silencing" or a shutdown of the added characteristic. A 1994 survey of thirty biotech companies showed that almost all had experienced gene silencing. A German study of genetically engineered petunias illustrates what can happen. Genetically engineered petunias were spliced with a corn gene to produce a salmon-red color. At the beginning of the season, 91 percent were strongly colored, 7.6 percent weakly colored. By the end of the season only 37 percent were strongly colored, and 60 percent weakly colored. These unexpected results show the instability with which newly introduced genes can switch on or off, and the effect the environment can have on the process.[7]

What might go wrong in the host organism with the arrival of the genetic cassette? (Keep in mind this is now the genetically modified organism or GMO.) Among other things, the cells in the GMO can begin to manufacture proteins in incorrect quantities or at the wrong times, and they can even begin to produce entirely new proteins. Put another way, genetically engineered foods may express or contain certain proteins, some of which are toxic to humans, in much higher levels than you are accustomed to eating, or they may contain entirely new foreign proteins, bacteria, or viral constructs that humans have never eaten before, either individually or in combination. In the worst-case scenario, gene-spliced foods can unexpectedly set off life-threatening food allergies or even poison you. (We'll have more to say about this in chapter 2.)

GENETIC ENGINEERING IS NOT JUST A SOUPED-UP VERSION OF TRADITIONAL AGRICULTURE

GENETIC ENGINEERING differs greatly from traditional crop breeding. Traditional crop breeding does not fundamentally alter or manipulate a plant's genes. Rather, it relies on the crossing or interbreeding of selected parents of the same or closely related species, using techniques of natural propagation such as pollination. The process of conventional breeding emphasizes certain characteristics—but those characteristics are not new to the species. As we know, humans can only mate with other humans; pigs can only mate with pigs. Corn can only pollinate with other strains of corn or closely related plant relatives.

In contrast, the process of genetically engineering foods involves using special chemical enzymes as scissors; extracting selected genes from a donor organism (i.e. animals, plants, insects, soil microorganisms, bacteria, and viruses); synthesizing or making copies of this genetic material, genetic promoters, and vectors; and then artificially inserting this synthetic "genetic cassette" into another completely different host organism, such as a soybean, a tomato, or a pig. The differences are not only in techniques and processes, but in the order of magnitude. Quite simply, genetic engineering goes far beyond the techniques of natural propagation, and brings new, untold risks.

GENETIC ENGINEERING: WHERE WILL IT LEAD US?

JUST BECAUSE the current gene-splicing capability of life science technicians utilizing gene guns and bacterial vectors is crude, inexact, and more or less unpredictable doesn't mean that the recombinant DNA technology of genetic engineering isn't "effective" in terms of giving birth to a living organism that is utterly new and "foreign." For example, when genes from humans are spliced into mice, pigs, or tobacco plants, the entire metabolism and "inner life" of these animals or plants begin to change.

COMING SOON TO THE BIOTECH CAFÉ

- Potatoes with jellyfish genes that glow when they need to be watered
- Super GE-enhanced salmon—twice as large as any salmon in history
- Vegetables with scorpion genes
- Pigs with human genes
- Tomatoes with flounder genes
- GE cows that produce human breast milk
- Corn plants or dairy products that contain pharmaceutical drugs
- Beer that can sit on the shelf for years
- Raw onions that won't make your eyes water
- Lemons in the shape of a star

FRANKENFOODS AND CROPS
LIVE ON . . . FOREVER

ONCE A living organism has been genetically engineered, its altered genetic codes begin to affect its internal and external life and chemical composition, altering every cell in the organism. This genetically engineered organism will then evolve and interact with its environment and other living organisms generation after generation, passing on its mutant characteristics, behavior, and imperfections to its offspring as well as to other related and unrelated organisms. In other words, GMOs have a life of their own. Like ordinary organisms they will genetically and chemically evolve in relation to changes in their environment, and they will pass these changes on to their offspring. In addition, they will exchange genetic material and thereby biochemical characteristics with related and even unrelated organisms in their environment.

For this reason, GMOs, once created and released into the environment, are permanent. They can never be recalled back into the laboratory, nor can they be contained within a restricted pasture, farmland, watershed, marine environment, or geographical space. Genetically engineered organisms are alive, mobile, and self-propagating. Like Frankenstein, once created and released from the laboratory, these living organisms cannot be tamed or killed. Frankenfoods and crops will live and mutate forever.

GENETIC DISINFORMATION:
MYTHS OF GENETICALLY
ENGINEERED FOODS & CROPS

BESIDES THE preposterous—and hazardous—scientific claim that gene-splicing is natural and that GE foods are "substantially equivalent" to conventional foods, the promoters of gene-foods and their allies in the food industry continue to publicize and promote the benefits of agricultural biotechnology. It is worth taking a closer look at some of the more problematic assertions made by the proponents of genetic engineering.

MYTH #1: GENE-SPLICING AND GENETIC ENGINEERING ARE PRECISE AND THERE-FORE GMOS ARE PREDICTABLE AND SAFE.

FACT: GENE-SPLICING is not a highly precise method of transferring genetic materials across species barriers. When shooting a gene-coated pellet at hundreds of miles an hour into the host organism, or using a bacterial vector, scientists have no way of knowing where the inserted foreign DNA will penetrate the cell chromosome, nor what will be the unintended consequences. Scientists understand very little about the biological function of most of the genetic material or DNA in plants, animals, and humans. Geneticists use the term "junk DNA" to describe the 97 percent of genetic material whose role in living organisms is not yet understood. Research in genetics tells us that individual genes do not operate in isolation, whereby one gene causes one, and only one, biological trait and gives rise to a uniform pattern of biochemical activity; rather, genes interact in a complex manner, changing their behavior in relation to influences from other genes in their own organism as well as being affected by other living organisms in their environment.

MYTH #2: GENETICALLY ENGINEERED FOODS HAVE INCREASED NUTRITIONAL VALUE.

FACT: ALTHOUGH genetic engineering companies have been promising us a cornucopia of more nutritious foods for almost two decades, no GE food currently on the market has been shown to be more nutritious or to taste better than non-GE foods. All of the four GE crops currently under commercial cultivation—soybeans, corn, canola, and cotton—have been genetically altered to express only two traits: to survive being sprayed with specific highly toxic broad-spectrum herbicides, or to produce their own insecticide, a toxin called Bt (*Bacillus thuringiensis*). In fact, certain GE foods have been shown to have less nutritional value and quality than conventional or non-GE foods (see chapter 2 for more details).

MYTH #3: GE CROPS WILL REDUCE THE USE OF TOXIC HERBICIDES AND PESTICIDES BY FARMERS.

FACT: THE manufacturers of genetically engineered seeds make enormous profits from selling toxic pesticides to farmers. The reason they are pushing herbicide-resistant GE crop seeds is so that they can sell more of their own broad-spectrum herbicides (which kill everything green except for herbicide-resistant GE plants) to farmers, not less.

According to a recent study based upon USDA government statistics, farmers using genetically engineered seeds on 550 million acres of crop land in the U.S. in 1996–2003 used 48 million additional pounds of pesticides than they would have used had they planted conventional or non-GE crops.[8] It's worth repeating that organic farmers—who are prohibited worldwide from using genetically engineered seeds or inputs—use no toxic pesticides or herbicides whatsoever.

As Dr. Charles Benbrook, Dr. Michael Hansen, and others point out in the book *Pest Management at the Crossroads,* the only real way to reduce pesticide use is through organic or sustainable agriculture practices—practices that include integrated pest management, crop rotation, cover crops, beneficial insects, planting a variety of crops, organic composting, manual/mechanical weeding, and natural bio-pesticides.

MYTH #4: FARMERS BENEFIT ECONOMICALLY FROM GROWING GE CROPS BECAUSE OF INCREASED YIELDS AND REDUCED INPUT COSTS.

FACT: FARMERS do not benefit economically from growing GE crops for a number of reasons. USDA government statistics for 1996–2003 show that farmers growing GE crops did not have overall yield or production increases. In fact, Dr. Charles Benbrook, former chair of the National Research Council's Agriculture Committee, has shown that farmers growing Monsanto's Roundup Ready soybeans—the most popular GE crop, comprising over 70 percent of all global acreage for GE crops—actually experienced yield decreases of approximately 7 percent in comparison to farmers who planted conventional soybeans.[9] In addition, GE seeds are more expensive than traditional seed varieties and often do not offer benefits that outweigh the extra cost. A study by Dr. Benbrook found that from 1996–2001, American farmers paid at least $659 million in price premiums to plant genetically engineered Bt corn, while boosting their harvest by only 276 million bushels—worth some $567 million in economic gain. The bottom line for farmers is a net loss of $92 million—about $1.31 per acre.[10] Moreover, beginning in 1999, major grain buyers in the U.S. such as Archer Daniels Midland and A.E. Staley began paying farmers a premium for growing non-GE crops. Because of strong opposition to GE foods in Europe, American farmers lost approximately $814 million in sales of corn exports in 1998–2003,[11] while soybean exports to the EU fell by over a billion dollars between 1996–99.[12]

With more and more overseas buyers in Europe and Japan demanding guaranteed non-GE foods, the American Corn Growers Association has warned farmers that they risk economic ruin by continuing to plant GE crop varieties. And because of unprecedented risks associated with GE crops, insurance companies in the U.S. and Europe are now reluctant to issue crop insurance policies on them.

MYTH #5: GENETICALLY ENGINEERED CROPS WILL FEED THE WORLD'S HUNGRY AND SAVE THE DEVELOPING WORLD FROM FAMINE.

FACT: ACCORDING to United Nations Food and Agriculture Organization, approximately 842 million people—out of a global population of over six billion—are chronically undernourished. This is a tragedy, as well as a moral and political outrage. But also according to the UN, the fundamental cause of world hunger is not a shortage of food in the world—in fact, there are immense surpluses—but rather that these 842 million hungry people are too poor to produce or buy the food that they need.

In fact, the world today produces more food per inhabitant than at any time in human history. The real causes of hunger are poverty, inequality, and lack of access to food.[13] Genetically engineered foods do nothing to address these root causes.

Additionally, genetically engineered technology is designed to make money. The technology allows the seed company to control the seed and pest control systems, all the while locking farmers into tough contracts to lease the technology. The technology takes away farmers' rights to grow their own food, save and improve their seed varieties, and help their community become more sustainable.

According to a number of scientific estimates, the world population is expected to level off and stabilize in approximately 50 years. At that time, analysts predict that there will still be ample food to feed us all, assuming people have the money they need to produce and/or buy their own food. But as research indicates the best and most sustainable way to produce an abundant and healthy global food supply will be to convert high-chemical and energy-intensive industrial farming—a major, if not *the* major contributing factor to global warming and climate change—into a system of sustainable and organic agriculture.

MYTH #6: THERE IS NO EVIDENCE THAT GE FOODS AND CROPS ARE HARMFUL TO HUMAN HEALTH OR TO THE ENVIRONMENT.

FACT: IN the next two chapters, we will take a close look at the mounting scientific evidence that genetically engineered foods and crops pose serious risks to human health, animals, and the environment. On May 17, 1999, the prestigious 115,000-member British Medical Association issued a report that called for a moratorium on GE foods and crops, declaring that more "independent" research is needed to determine the possible toxicity of bioengineered food. The BMA warned that the commercialization of untested and unlabeled gene-foods could lead to the development of new allergies and antibiotic resistance in humans.

On December 14, 1999, 231 scientists from 31 countries published an "Open Letter to All Governments" calling for a global moratorium on all genetically engineered foods and crops. In the text the scientists call for "the immediate suspension of all environmental releases of genetically modified crops and products; for patents on life-forms and living processes to be revoked and banned; and for a comprehensive public enquiry into the future of agriculture and food security for all." The scientists note specifically that the "cauliflower mosaic viral promoter, widely used in genetically modified crops, may enhance horizontal gene transfer and has the potential to generate new viruses that cause diseases."

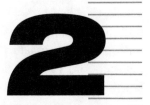

WHAT ARE THE HUMAN HEALTH RISKS OF GENETICALLY ENGINEERED FOODS?

GENETICALLY ENGINEERED products clearly have the potential to be toxic and a threat to human health. But exactly what are the threats? And how serious are they? When looking at the potential human health impacts of consuming genetically engineered foods, what jumps out are the startling number of questions that thus far have been left unanswered. There still continue to be no long-term feeding studies (traditionally done with laboratory animals) to gain insight into what effects many of the commonly consumed genetically engineered foods might have on our health. A short-term feeding study carried out with human volunteers in the UK in 2002 indicated that a major proportion of genetically modified DNA survived passage through the small intestine, allowing antibiotic-resistant marker genes to recombine with bacteria commonly found in the human gut.[1] The concern here, of course, is that dangerous bacteria will develop a resistance to antibiotics, making it difficult for doctors to treat some human illnesses. For these and other reasons, the British Medical Association and a growing number of independent scientists have called for a moratorium on genetically engineered foods until further research is completed.

Without strong data supporting safety, we are left to look at the research and case studies that have been completed—and thus far, this growing body of evidence indicates that genetically engineered food may cause toxic effects, exposure to allergens, and elevated cancer risks. As you will see in this chapter, genetic engineering is already associated with one deadly disaster in 1988, which killed thirty-seven people, and a near-disaster related to a food allergen in 1996. Additionally, the only thorough independent feeding study of genetically engineered foods, carried out with genetically engineered potatoes at the Rowett Research Institute in Scotland in 1996–98, produced serious adverse effects in rats—setting off alarm bells around the world.

In the end, we are left with more questions than answers. And more concerns than confidence. Let's examine in more detail what we do know.

THE L-TRYPTOPHAN DISASTER: A WARNING OF THINGS TO COME?

ONE OF the major concerns with genetically engineered foods is that the process of genetic engineering is itself unstable, inexact, and prone to mistakes with potentially fatal consequences. A cautionary tale of genetic engineering gone wrong is the story of L-tryptophan.

In the late 1980s, a genetically engineered brand of L-tryptophan, a common over-the-counter nutritional supplement used to treat insomnia and depression, killed 37 Americans and permanently disabled or afflicted more than 5,000 others with a potentially fatal and painful blood disorder called eosinophilia myalgia syndrome (EMS). Reacting to the tragedy, the Food and Drug Administration (FDA) pulled L-tryptophan off the market. Thousands of EMS victims suffered, and continue to suffer, from a wide variety of painful and life-threatening symptoms including heart disease, severe muscle pain, memory loss, and paralysis.[2]

The manufacturer, Showa Denko K.K., Japan's third largest chemical company, had for the first time in the late-1980s used genetically engineered bacteria to increase the efficiency of tryptophan production by inserting genes that caused the bacteria to express new enzymes.[3] Safety tests of the new gene-altered L-tryptophan were not required by the U.S. FDA because the tryptophan produced by non-genetically engineered bacteria had been sold for years without ill effects, and the FDA assumed that GE and non-GE L-tryptophan were "substantially equivalent." Instead, it is believed that the bacteria somehow became contaminated during the recombinant (gene-splicing) DNA process.

The FDA and Showa Denko at first suggested that "inadequate purification," rather than genetic engineering, was the cause of the tragedy. But Showa Denko's own lawyer, Richard Hinds, argued in court that the chemical filtering process was not to blame.[4] Showa Denko has already paid out $1 billion in damages to EMS victims. Neither Showa Denko, the FDA, the biotechnology industry, nor the nutritional supplement industry have ever carried out an in-depth, scientifically rigorous analysis of the deadly incident.

PUSZTAI'S POTATOES:
INDICTING ALL GENE-SPLICED FOODS?

INDEPENDENT SCIENTIFIC research on genetically engineered foods is rare, particularly research that studies the possible adverse effects of consuming such foods. Traditionally, the scientific community does not treat humans as guinea pigs by feeding them new food or drug products. Instead, rats are commonly used as a surrogate in feeding studies.

One of the few instances of independent research involving rat feeding of genetically engineered foods was carried out by Dr. Arpad Pusztai and a team of researchers at the prestigious Rowett Institute in Scotland in the late 1990s Pusztai's research team, highly regarded by the biotechnology industry and the British government, won out over more than a dozen other biotech labs in a competition to secure a multimillion dollar grant to study the potential impact of genetically engineered potatoes on animal and human health. What Dr. Pusztai, a self-described "proponent" of genetically engineered foods, found was so explosive that his research was the subject of numerous headline stories in the British press in late 1998 and early 1999.

Pusztai's research team found that GE pest-resistant potatoes, spliced with DNA from the snowdrop plant and a commonly used viral promoter (present in almost all gene-foods), the Cauliflower Mosaic Virus (CaMv), were apparently poisonous to laboratory rats. The implications of Pusztai's partially completed research studies were far-reaching and profoundly disturbing, because they seemed to indicate that:

- There are significant chemical and compositional differences between conventional and genetically engineered foods.
- There are significant nutritional variations or protein levels in different batches of the same GE food, likely caused by the inherent unpredictability of the gene-splicing process itself.
- There can be damage to the vital organs and immune systems of lab animals fed genetically engineered foods, in this case potatoes.
- There is evidence that the Cauliflower Mosaic Viral Promoter (CaMv), gene-spliced into almost all genetically engineered foods, may be harmful to lab animals, and therefore may be harmful to humans.

GE FOODS ARE DIFFERENT FROM
CONVENTIONAL FOODS

DR. PUSZTAI'S team found that potatoes gene-spliced with a substance having pest-resistant qualities called a lectin (transplanted in this case from the bulb of a snowdrop plant) were significantly different in chemical composition from conventional, non-GE potatoes.

Moreover, Pusztai found that GE potatoes were not only compositionally different from non-GE potatoes, but that, even among themselves, different batches of GE potatoes were significantly different. This finding of batch variation in GE varieties is also tremendously significant, since it underscores the inherent unpredictability of gene-spliced foods and reminds us just how incredibly difficult it will be to carry out reliable chemical and safety tests on these foods. As Pusztai explains:

"We had two transgenic lines of potato produced from the same gene insertion and the same growing conditions; we grew them together along with the parent plant. With our two lines of potato, which should have been substantially equivalent to each other, we found that one of the lines contained 20 percent less protein than the other. But we also found that these two lines were not substantially equivalent to their parent. This could not be predicted. It demonstrates that the unpredictability is inherent in the GM (genetic modification) process on a case-by-case basis and also at the level of every single GM plant created."[5]

GE POTATOES POISONED RATS

BESIDES SIGNIFICANT compositional differences, Pusztai found that, after only ten days, the gene-spliced potatoes damaged the vital organs and immune systems of lab rats, whereas rats fed conventional potatoes, and rats fed conventional potatoes with lectin added mechanically (with an eye-dropper), as opposed to lectin added genetically (i.e. through gene-splicing), were unharmed. This research strongly suggests that it is not the foreign protein itself (the snowdrop lectin DNA in this case) that is poisonous—otherwise the rats that ate the potatoes with the lectin added mechanically would have been harmed—but rather something inherent in the gene-splicing process itself.

QUESTIONS ABOUT ALTERED VIRUSES IN GENE-FOODS

PERHAPS MOST alarming of all, Pusztai and Dr. Stanley Ewen, a pathologist at the University of Aberdeen in Scotland, drew the interim conclusion that damage to the rats' intestines and stomach linings—apparently a severe viral infection—most likely was caused by the CaMv viral promoter, a promoter derived from the Cauliflower Mosaic Virus, which is gene-spliced as a chemical switch into nearly all GE foods and crops. As Pusztai noted in an article in the U.K. Sunday Herald, "If there really is a problem [with the CaMv viral promoter], it probably won't apply just to the potatoes, but probably to all other transgenes [i.e. all other GE foods]."[6] In other words every gene-food out there containing the CaMv viral promoter could have unknown effects on our organs and immune system.

Many other scientists from around the world have echoed Dr. Pusztai's warnings about the inherent dangers of genetically engineered foods and the use of the Cauliflower Mosaic Viral Promoter. Dr. Mae-Wan Ho, Angela Ryan, and Dr. Joe Cummins (no relation to the coauthor), researchers at The Open University in England and University of Western Ontario, Canada, highlight human health risks associated with the CaMv: "The use of the Cauliflower Mosaic Viral promoter (CaMv) has the potential to reactivate dormant viruses or create new viruses in all species to which it is transferred. This transgenic instability increases the possibility of promotion of an inappropriate over-expression of genes to the transferred species. The development of cancer may be one consequence of such inappropriate over-expression of genes." Ho, Ryan, and Cummins strongly recommend that all transgenic crops and animal feeds containing CaMv be banned.[7]

UNFINISHED BUSINESS

DR. PUSZTAI'S pathbreaking research work on GE potatoes unfortunately remains incomplete. Government funding was cut off, and he was fired and locked out of his lab after he spoke to the British media about his concerns over the dangers of GE foods.[8] As Joel Bleifuss reported in the January 10, 2000, issue of *In These Times* magazine, Pusztai's research, especially after he published an article in the prestigious British medical journal *Lancet* in October 1999, threatened the powerful biotech scientific establishment:

"The condemnation from the pro-genetic engineering scientific establishment was immediate. The Royal Society accused the *Lancet* of being 'breathtakingly arrogant' for publishing Pusztai's research. The *Guardian* (a leading U.K. newspaper) reported that two days before the publication of the Pusztai paper, *Lancet* editor Richard Horton had been warned by a senior member of the Royal Society . . . that his job would be in jeopardy if he published Pusztai's research."[9]

But as we have noted, more and more scientists around the world have rallied to Pusztai's defense, warning that the genetic engineering of the common foods that you and your family eat everyday may be hazardous. Vilified by the pro-biotech establishment, Dr. Pusztai will nonetheless go down in history as a scientific hero, a genetic engineer who dared to speak the truth even though it cost him his job and possibly his career as a research scientist.[10]

THE NEAR-DISASTER OF GE SOYBEANS:
ARE GENE-FOODS ALLERGENIC?

WHENEVER A new food product is introduced into the food supply, one of the first safety screens is whether it contains any known allergens. In conventional foods this process is as simple as looking at the ingredients. But genetically engineered foods pose unique challenges and questions. Are known allergens spliced into gene foods possible food allergens? And what about the introduction of new proteins never before consumed by humans? How do we determine that these new proteins are not allergenic? The research done thus far indicates that the potential exposure to food allergens is a very real concern when it comes to GE foods.

When University of Nebraska researchers reported their findings on March 14, 1996, in the *New England Journal of Medicine* it suddenly raised the stakes in the new world of genetically engineered foods. The Nebraska researchers found that Brazil nut DNA, gene-spliced into conventional soybeans, could induce potentially fatal allergies in people sensitive to Brazil nuts. The company preparing to mass market the Brazil nut-spliced soybeans, Pioneer Hi-Bred (now owned by Dupont), immediately ceased plans for production. Pioneer had hoped to market the GE soybeans, containing elevated levels of an amino acid called methionine (found in Brazil nuts, but contained only in very low levels in conventional soybeans), as a more nutritious animal feed.[11]

While Pioneer Hi-Bred scientists had characterized their research on the GE soybeans as "very promising," the *Washington Post* had declared in 1992: "Because brazil nuts and methionine are known to be safe, the new soybean variety might not require formal FDA approval."[12] In addition, animal feeding tests of these Brazil nut–spliced soybeans, usually not even required before placing GE foods on the market, had turned up negative when looking at allergenicity. According to Dr. Steve Taylor, the University of Nebraska researcher who discovered the allergenicity of the Pioneer Hi-Bred soybeans, the failure of animal feeding tests to uncover the potentially life-threatening allergenicity of the elevated levels of methionine in the gene-altered beans "emphasizes why we cannot rely exclusively on animal-based tests for these determinations."[13] Unfortunately, the U.S. government does not require the kind of human allergy testing that Dr. Taylor performed—which in this case prevented a potential public health disaster.

STARLINK CORN: AMERICA'S LARGEST GE FOOD RECALL

ON SEPTEMBER 18, 2000, American consumers were shocked by media reports that an illegal, likely allergenic variety of genetically engineered corn, called StarLink, had contaminated over 300 brand-name food products, including taco shells, corn meal, and corn chips—resulting in a massive recall of millions of packaged foods. Over the next month several hundred U.S. consumers complained to the FDA that they had suffered allergic reactions after consuming products likely containing StarLink corn, reactions which ranged all the way from mild unpleasantness to severe shock. Although StarLink had been planted in only about one percent of America's cornfields (312,000 acres), after routine comingling and mixing in grain silos, railroad cars, barges, and truck shipments, it eventually contaminated over 20 percent of all corn tested by the USDA.[14] Although the FDA was not able to confirm that StarLink had indeed caused allergic reactions in consumers, Aventis, the company that developed StarLink, voluntarily pulled it off the market. This action enabled Aventis to avoid some of the legal and public relations fallout from a formal government ban on the corn.

The StarLink scandal made headlines, generated thousands of news articles and TV clips, and brought home the realization to U.S. consumers that the nation's supermarkets are filled with an extensive inventory of untested, unlabeled genetically engineered foods. StarLink was produced by gene-splicing a powerful soil bacteria called Bt (bacillus thuringiensis) into corn. Developed by AgrEvo, a subsidiary of the French-German biotech conglomerate Aventis (now owned by Bayer), StarLink was approved for cultivation by the EPA in 1998, but only for animal feed, because of fears that this particular Cry9c variety (50–100 times more potent than other Bt-spliced corn varieties) might set off serious food allergies. Subsequently it turned out that not only was StarLink not safety-tested before it was put on the market, but that the FDA had relied entirely on the company's own safety assessment, as it does for all GE crops and foods.[15] According to the *Washington Post*: "StarLink is suspected of causing allergies because Cry9c has a heightened ability to resist heat and gastric juices—giving more time for the body to overreact."[16] Although the EPA was supposed to require that Starlink's parent company tell farmers that they had to keep StarLink separate from corn destined for the human feed chain, most farmers said they were unaware of this requirement and had taken no special precautions. In 2003, three years after the StarLink crisis, the USDA was still finding traces of StarLink corn in export shipments.

As the StarLink debacle unfolded, America's overseas customers refused all corn export shipments, costing farmers and grain companies hundreds of millions of dollars in lost sales, while EPA and USDA officials scrambled to assure consumers at home and abroad that this type of incident would not happen again. Although consumer alarm over StarLink subsided after a few months, the incident served to demonstrate that once genetically engineered crops like corn are grown outside of the laboratory, comingling and contamination are very difficult, if not impossible, to prevent. Underlining this threat, the government was forced to admit two years later, in 2002, that an even more dangerous variety of GE corn, spliced with pharmaceutical drugs, had likewise contaminated millions of pounds of corn and soybeans in Nebraska and Iowa.

THE THREAT OF UNKNOWN ALLERGIES

THE CENTERS for Disease Control estimate that 2 percent of all adults and 8 percent of all children suffer from food allergies, whose symptoms can range from mild unpleasantness to sudden death. According to the Consumers Union, medical polls show that 25 percent of Americans report that they or members of their families suffer from food allergies or sensitivities.

An increasing number of scientists are concerned that the new proteins spliced into genetically engineered foods could be allergenic. As Dr. Rebecca Goldburg of the public interest group Environmental Defense states, "Since genetic engineers mix genes from a wide variety of species. . . . People who are allergic to one type of food may find that they are allergic to many more."[17]

In a Consumers International position paper, "Why We Need Labeling of Genetically Engineered Food," Jean Halloran and Dr. Michael Hansen warn that: "Proteins are what cause allergic reactions, and virtually every gene transfer in crops results in some protein production. Proteins will be coming into food crops not just from known sources of food allergens, like peanuts, shellfish, and dairy, but from plants of all kinds, bacteria, and viruses, whose potential allergenicity is uncommon or unknown."

Allergies caused by genetically engineered foods are extremely difficult to predict in advance. There are no 100 percent accurate tests for newly introduced proteins to find out whether they will be allergic in humans. "We all wish there was a test where you plug in a protein and out pops a 'yes' or 'no' answer," says Sue MacIntosh, a protein chemist with the biotech company AgrEvo.[18]

Unfortunately animal feeding studies, as the Pioneer Brazil nut–spliced soybean case graphically illustrates, may not be adequate to find out whether particular gene-foods are likely to give you health-damaging or life-threatening food allergies. And of course these types of animal feeding tests are not even required by the government, except in those rare cases where known allergens such as peanuts or shellfish are being gene-spliced into a common food.

Only long-term volunteer human feeding studies could even begin to tell us if gene-foods are allergenic. These volunteer human feeding studies would have to be conducted on a long-term basis since human food allergies are known to build up over time. But as we've pointed out, volunteer human allergy studies are currently not required before GE companies commercialize gene-foods. As the *New England Journal of Medicine* warned in its March 14, 1996, issue regarding "foreign proteins" being gene-spliced into common food products: "The allergenic potential of these newly introduced microbial proteins is uncertain, unpredictable, and untestable."[19]

There are new concerns that GE crops could also cause allergic reactions in farmworkers. In February 2004 Norwegian scientist Terje Traavik released a study that found that Philippine farmers living near GE corn fields were suffering from allergic reactions to drifting corn pollen, causing a range of symptoms including "fevers and respiratory, intestinal, and skin ailments."[20]

ARE GE-INDUCED ALLERGIES ALREADY DAMAGING YOUR HEALTH?

EUROPEAN FEARS over increased human allergies from genetically engineered foods increased substantially after an article in the U.K.'s *Daily Express* (March 12, 1999) reported that scientists at the York Nutritional Laboratory in Britain found an unusual 50 percent increase in food allergies from Britons' ingesting soy products in 1998, coinciding with a major increase in GE soybean imports from the U.S. According to the *Express*, "Researchers at the York Nutritional Laboratory said their findings provide real evidence that GM food could have a tangible, harmful impact on the human body." John Graham, spokesman for the York laboratory, said: "We believe this raises serious new questions about the safety of GM foods. . . . It is the first time in seventeen years of testing that soy has crept into the laboratory's top ten foods to cause an allergic reaction in consumers."

British scientists have expressed concerns about the potential allergenic quality of genetically engineered soybeans for several years. British biotech expert Dr. Mae-Won Ho, among others, has warned that Monsanto's RoundupReady soybeans could pose serious food allergy problems. As Dr. Ho stated in a legal affidavit in August 1998, Monsanto's RR soybeans "contain genes from a virus, a soil bacterium and from a petunia (plant), none of which have been in our food before. . . . The soil bacterium, Agrobacterium sp. (CP4EPSPS) . . . is unlike any other protein that humans have eaten. And there is no reliable method for predicting its allergenic potential. Allergic reactions typically occur only some time after the subject is sensitized by initial exposure to the allergen.[21]

RECOMBINANT BOVINE GROWTH HORMONE (RBGH) AND CANCER RISKS

UTILIZING GENETIC engineering for animals poses unique problems—both for the animals and humans. The best known, and in many ways the most alarming, genetic alteration of the U.S. food supply centers around a genetically engineered hormone called recombinant Bovine Growth Hormone (rBGH), sometimes known as rBST. Approved for sale by the FDA in February 1994, rBGH is injected into dairy cows to force them to produce 10–15 percent more milk. The government approved rBGH, the world's first GE food product, even though scientists from the Consumers Union and the Cancer Prevention Coalition warned that significantly higher levels of a potent chemical hormone, Insulin-Like Growth Factor (IGF-1), in the milk and dairy products of injected cows, could pose serious hazards for human breast, prostate, and colon cancer. A number of studies have shown that humans with elevated levels of IGF-1 in their bodies are much more likely to get cancer and that IGF-1 is a powerful cancer tumor promoter.[22]

Dr. Samuel Epstein, Professor of Environmental Medicine at

the University of Illinois School of Public Health, summarized the cancer and other human health hazards of rBGH in a British magazine, *The Ecologist* (September–October 1998): "[Recombinant Bovine Growth Hormone] differs from natural milk chemically, nutritionally, pharmacologically, and immunologically, besides being contaminated with pus and antibiotics resulting from mastitis induced by the biotech hormone. rBGH has high levels of abnormally potent IGF-1, up to ten times the levels in natural milk and over ten times more potent. IGF-1 resists pasteurization and digestion by stomach enzymes and is well absorbed across the intestinal wall. Still-unpublished Monsanto tests, disclosed by the FDA in summary form in 1990, showed that statistically significant growth-stimulating effects were induced in organs of adult rats by feeding IGF-1 at the lowest dose levels for only two weeks. Drinking rBGH milk would thus be expected to increase blood IGF-1 levels and to increase risks of developing prostate cancer and promoting its invasiveness. Multiple lines of evidence have also incriminated the role of IGF-1 as risk factors for breast, colon, and childhood cancers . . ."

In other words, you should be very concerned about whether or not the milk and dairy products you and your family consume are coming from cows injected with rBGH because:

- The milk from rBGH-injected cows has much higher levels of a powerful growth hormone factor called IGF-1, which is a potent cancer tumor promoter.
- rBGH-injected cows, according to the Consumers Union, have much higher rates of udder infections, called mastitis, which are routinely treated by injecting the animals with powerful antibiotics, some of which—in a nation like the U.S. where there is inadequate monitoring of antibiotic residues—inevitably end up as residues in your milk and other dairy products, not to mention in your hamburger meat.
- rBGH milk, according to Epstein and the Consumers Union, contains higher levels of pus and bacteria.

Underlining these concerns, the U.S. Congressional watchdog agency the Government Accounting Office basically told the FDA in 1993 not to approve rBGH, arguing that the probability of increased antibiotic residues in the milk of rBGH-injected cows (resulting from higher rates of udder infections among rBGH-injected cows) posed an unacceptable risk for public health. What this means is that if you routinely ingest antibiotic animal drug residues in the meat, dairy products, and milk you consume, over time your body can become resistant to antibiotics—a serious problem in the U.S. (as this chapter will later detail). Then if you become seriously ill and need antibiotics, they may not work.

MONSANTO'S RAT FEEDING STUDIES: THE SMOKING GUN?

IN 1998, government scientists in Canada released heretofore undisclosed Monsanto/FDA documents showing damage to laboratory rats fed dosages of rBGH. Significant infiltration of rBGH into the prostate of the rats as well as thyroid cysts indicated potential cancer hazards from the drug.[23] Subsequently the government of Canada, under heavy pressure from consumers, banned rBGH in early 1999. The European Union essentially has had a ban in place since 1993. Although rBGH continues to be injected into approximately 20 percent of all U.S. dairy cows, no other industrialized countries, except for Mexico and Brazil, have legalized its use. The GATT Codex Alimentarius, a United Nations food standards body, has refused to certify that rBGH is safe. Even though 74 percent of Americans stated in a USDA-funded poll published in 1996 that they believe rBGH poses hazards for human health, U.S. regulatory agencies have refused to take the drug off the market, or even to require mandatory labeling for dairy products derived from rBGH-injected cows.[24] Later in this book we'll tell you how to find milk, beef, and dairy products that do not come from cows injected with rBGH.

WHEN GENE engineers splice a foreign protein into a food prod-uct, they most often link it to another gene, called an antibiotic-resistance marker (ARM) gene. By dousing this new genetically engineered creation with an antibiotic, the genetic engineer can tell if the gene-splicing procedure was successful. Basically, if the antibiotic doesn't kill the gene-food, the splicing was successful, since the inserted antibiotic-resistant marker gene provided pro-tection. This all sounds clever, but unfortunately there is a down-side to ARM-ing genes.

What is worrisome to scientists and public health officials is the possibility or likelihood that ARM genes employed in gene-spliced foods or animal feeds may "mate" or combine with an expanded range of preexisting germs or pathogens and give rise to deadly new strains of antibiotic resistant "superbugs" (salmonella, E. coli, campylobacter, tuberculosis, staph, and enterococcus).

ARMed genes may be contributing factors to the growing public health problem of infections that cannot be cured with ampicillin, kanamycin, penicillin, or other traditional antibiotics. This phenom-enon of inadvertently transferring antibiotic resistance into non-tar-get organisms or pathogens is one of the prime examples of what is called "horizontal gene transfer"—a phenomena that was extremely rare in nature until the advent of genetic engineering. Geneticists call this type of "unnatural" genetic transmission "horizontal gene transfer" to differentiate it from the normal "vertical gene transfer" that occurs when non-genetically engineered living organisms pass their genes and genetic characteristics on to their offspring.

Dutch scientists found, in a sophisticated computer simulation of the human digestive system, that ARM genes in genetically engineered food could recombine with bacteria already present in the human gut to give rise to new strains of bacteria. "The results show that DNA lingers in the intestine, and confirms that geneti-cally modified bacteria can transfer their antibiotic resistance genes to bacteria in the gut," the Dutch scientists reported in *New Scientist* magazine.[25]

This computer simulation was confirmed in a 2002 feeding study in the U.K. at Newcastle University in which seven human volunteers were fed soy burgers and soy milk containing genetically engineered soybeans, including antibiotic-resistant marker genes.[26] Researchers found that the ARM genes survived digestion in the small intestine, transferring antibiotic resistance to the bacteria found in the gut of the human volunteers. This study, according to British scientist Dr. Michael Antoniou, is extremely important: "Everyone used to deny that this was possible. It suggests that you can get antibiotic marker genes spreading around the stomach, which would compromise antibiotic resistance. They have shown that this can happen even at very low levels after just one meal."[27]

In another study, British scientists found that ARMs and other transgenic DNA can recombine with bacteria in the human mouth and throat for up to an hour after being ingested, thereby giving rise to new strains of bacteria.[28] Given the emerging science on ARMs it comes as no surprise that the respected British Medical Association warned as early as 1999 that the use of antibiotic-resistant marker genes "should be phased out as swiftly as possible." European authorities are currently considering a ban on all GE foods containing antibiotic resistant marker genes, and have begun to implement a ban on antibiotics added to animal feeds.

GE VECTORS AND VIRAL PROMOTERS: ARE WE CREATING A GLOBAL HOT ZONE?

YOU'VE UNDOUBTEDLY seen or heard about Hollywood movies like *Outbreak* or *The Hot Zone* or watched the television show *X-Files*. These and a similar genre of mass-market paperbacks are scary enough to be science fiction, but many of them in fact are based upon real world events. New deadly viral- and bacterial-based diseases are emerging with greater and greater frequency across the world. One need only consider the emergence and global devastation of the AIDS virus—a virus that inexplicably jumped from monkeys to humans sometime over the last few decades—to become alarmed about emerging infectious diseases. On the bacterial and food safety front, the mysterious appearance in 1982 of the E. coli 0157:H7 pathogen, the "hamburger disease" has likewise caused fear and consternation, with 60,000 Americans yearly being poisoned by the food-borne bacterium, including fifty-two reported deaths in 1998. The U.S. Department of Agriculture recently admitted that over 50 percent of U.S. beef carcasses are now contaminated with E. coli 0157:H7.[29] A number of scientists, including Dr. Mae-Won Ho from the U.K. and Dr. Terje Traavik from Norway, have warned that the dumping of increasing amounts of genetically engineered vectors, viral promoters, and ARM genes into the environment may be inadvertently causing new super-virulent viruses and bacteria to cross traditional species barriers and threaten human health.[30]

INCREASED PESTICIDE RESIDUES ON FOODS

AS WE noted previously, contrary to biotech industry claims, recent studies have found that U.S. farmers growing GE crops are typically using more, not less, toxic pesticides and herbicides than conventional farmers—48 million more pounds from 1996–2003, in fact.[31] Scientists also predict that as weeds and pests inevitably develop resistance to GE crops, even more herbicides and pesticides will be used. There is certainly no doubt that farmers growing GE crops are using more super-potent "broad-spectrum" herbicides such as glyphosate (Roundup), glufosinate, and bromoxynil than ever before. Crops genetically engineered to be resistant to broad-spectrum herbicides accounted for approximately 75 percent of all global GE crops planted in 2003.

The so-called "benefit" of herbicide-resistant crops is that farmers can spray as much of a particular company's herbicide on their crops as they want—killing the weeds without killing their crop. Broad-spectrum herbicides, used in conjunction with herbicide-resistant seeds, are designed to literally kill everything green. Farmers like the Roundup Ready crops because they consider Roundup less toxic than what they normally use. Monsanto and other companies estimate that herbicide-resistant crops planted around the globe will triple the amount of toxic broad-spectrum herbicides used in agriculture.

A number of recent scientific studies have linked these super weed-killers to increased risks for cancer, birth defects, and other health hazards. In a 1999 article in the medical research journal *Cancer* (Volume 86 (6)), foods with residues of glyphosate, the active ingredient in Monsanto's top-selling broad spectrum herbicide, Roundup, commonly used in herbicide-resistant crops such as soybeans, corn, cotton, and canola, are cited as possible hazards for an increasingly common form of cancer, non-Hodgkin's lymphoma.[32] Laboratory studies have shown that glyphosate causes a wide range of adverse health reactions, even at low doses. Animals fed glyphosate have experienced reduced weight gain, diarrhea, salivary gland lesions, liver damage, cataracts, and increases in thyroid, pancreas, and liver tumors. Glyphosate has also been observed to cause genetic damage in human blood cells, fruit flies, and onion cells.[33] In September 2003 Denmark implemented a partial ban on the spraying of glyphosate, after alarming levels of the herbicide turned up in the drinking water of Copenhagen and other cities. Officials blamed the drinking water contamination on farmers' repeated spraying of the Roundup herbicide.[34]

PESTICIDE RESIDUES IN YOUR SHOPPING CART

IN 1996, as increasing amounts of Roundup herbicide began to be sprayed on GE crops in North America, government regulatory officials in the EU raised the legal daily limit of glyphosate residues that can be ingested by humans to 20 mg per kilo—sixty times greater than the "acceptable daily intake" level previously recommended by the World Health Organization. In a similar move, Environmental Protection Agency officials in the U.S. had previously raised legally acceptable glyphosate intake levels to 100 mg per kilo—ten times the level at which birth and reproductive abnormalities have been observed in mammals.[35] In 1998 over 112,000 tons of glyphosate, the world's largest selling herbicide, were sprayed across the globe. What this means is that you might be getting more than you bargained for in your soyburger, in your tofu, in your baby food, and in the thousands of other supermarket foods that now contain GE soy or soy-derived ingredients.

Increased herbicide use on animal feed crops means that increased residues (on soybean hulls for example) in animal feeds will end up concentrating in the fatty tissues of these animals. Dr. Marc Lappe, author of the 1998 book, *Against the Grain*, points out that "Use of herbicide tolerant crops virtually guarantees that beef, poultry, and pork will have higher contamination levels of such pesticides than livestock had previously," and that government allowances of significantly higher pesticide residues will expose consumers, especially infants and children, to a "largely untested and different burden of pesticides than before."[36] The bottom line for meat-eaters is that that you're probably ingesting record amounts of Roundup pesticide in your burgers, chicken, and bacon. That is, of course, unless you're buying "certified organic" products, which we discuss later in the book.

Roundup, though the most commonly used, is not the only broad-spectrum herbicide that is worrisome. Glufosinate, the active ingredient in a number of herbicide-resistant crops sold by Aventis, Monsanto, and other companies, has been linked to birth defects, learning disabilities, and abnormal behavior in the children of pregnant women who consumed foods (soybeans, corn, and canola oil) with glufosinate residues.[37] Even more alarming is the toxic weed-killer bromoxynil, manufactured by Aventis, sprayed in heavy doses on herbicide-resistant GE cotton plants (and ending up in cotton seed and vegetable oils), which even the EPA classifies as a "possible human carcinogen."[38] As Lappe reports in *Against the Grain*, bromoxynil has been linked with liver tumors, spinal and skull defects, reduced fetal weight, and developmental disorders in human fetuses.

PHARM CROPS: PHARMACEUTICAL DRUGS IN YOUR CORN FLAKES

AMONG THE most hazardous and unpredictable new products in the biotech pipeline are the so-called "pharm," or "biopharm" crops. These are crops, most often corn or tobacco, that are gene-spliced to produce powerful pharmaceutical drugs and industrial chemicals. Drug and chemical companies are excited about biopharming, since using plants or animals as "bioreactors" can reduce their manufacturing costs. The downside is that these mutant bioreactors may pollute the environment and contaminate the food chain.

Over the past few years more than 315 fields of biopharm crops have been planted in the U.S.—in secret locations in the open environment. Biopharm crops have been gene-spliced to produce human and animal vaccines, blood-clotting agents, abortion-inducing compounds, and other powerful drugs. Pharm crops have also been cultivated to produce plastics, industrial enzymes, synthetic fabrics, and other chemicals. Approximately 200 of these experiments have been conducted with corn, notorious for spreading its wind-blown pollen to surrounding fields. Although no pharm crops have been approved for commercial production, regulations and enforcement of test plots are notoriously lax.[39] Biopharm companies are not even required to give the USDA the exact gene sequences of the experimental crops, according to Dr. Michael Hansen of the Consumers Union, making it impossible for the government to verify whether or not particular pharm crops have contaminated the food chain. As Larry Bohlen of Friends of the Earth put it, "Just one mistake by a biotech company and we'll be eating other people's prescription drugs in our corn flakes."[40] Recent events indicate that this contamination is already taking place.

In November 2002 the USDA admitted that at least two experimental corn crops in Nebraska and Iowa, grown by ProdiGene, a biopharm company, had already polluted the environment. Not only had at least one, and possibly both, of the mutant corn crops pollinated, thereby spreading their mutant genes into the air, but several hundred "volunteer" ProdiGene corn plants had sprung up the following year, contaminating over 500,000 bushels of soybeans in Nebraska, and 150 acres of corn in Iowa.[41] ProdiGene at first tried to deny there was a problem, but then issued an apology. The USDA imposed $3 million in penalties on ProdiGene, but brushed off demands by public interest groups for a complete moratorium on biopharm experiments.[42]

According to USDA records and an FDA memo posted on the Web site of the Organic Consumers Association, ProdiGene holds permits to grow corn that has been genetically engineered to express a pig vaccine, as well as corn gene-spliced to produce a controversial AIDS drug called HIV glycoprotein gp120, a blood-clotting agent (aprotinin). ProdiGene, under pressure, admitted that some of the plants cited in their violation were designed to express a pig vaccine, but a November 2002 FDA memo strongly suggests that it was the AIDS drug or some other human drug—not the pig virus—that was being grown by ProdiGene in Nebraska.[43]

ProdiGene's biopharm blunder was the most serious biotech scandal since the StarLink controversy in 2000, when a likely allergenic variety of feed corn contaminated the U.S. food chain and generated major controversy in the press, both in the U.S. and worldwide. For the first time since the advent of GE foods and crops in 1994, major U.S. grocery store chains, represented by the Grocery Manufacturers of America, and food corporations, represented by the National Food Processors Association, clashed with the USDA and the biotech industry, demanding that biopharm companies stop experimenting with food and animal feed crops such as corn. Even the Biotechnology Industry Organization (BIO), the trade association for medical and agbiotech companies, briefly called for a moratorium on biopharm experiments in the Midwestern corn belt in October 2002. BIO reversed itself shortly thereafter, however, caving in to pressure from biotech and agribusiness lobbyists.

DAMAGE TO FOOD QUALITY & NUTRITION

DOES GENETICALLY engineered food have damaged vitamin content or nutritional value? This is a very important question for all consumers. Unfortunately, as the critics of gene-foods have pointed out, the U.S. government does not require stringent chemical and nutritional analyses of new genetically engineered foods before companies place these foods on the market.

Although very little research has been done on the damage of genetic engineering to food quality and nutrition, an important 1999 study by Dr. Marc Lappe published in the *Journal of Medicinal Food* found that concentrations of beneficial phyto-estrogen compounds, thought to protect against heart disease and cancer, were 12–14 percent lower in genetically modified soy-beans than in traditional soybean varieties. These and other studies, including Dr. Pusztai's, indicate that genetically engineering food may result in foods lower in protein quality, disease-fighting capabilities, and nutrition. For example the milk from cows injected with rBGH contains higher levels of pus, bacteria, and fat, while dairy cows ingesting GE soybeans have exhibited higher levels of fat in their milk, as reported in a study released by Greenpeace International in October 1997.

Unfortunately, serious questions about the toxicity, allergenicity, cancer risks, and nutritional content of genetically engineered foods remain unanswered.[44] This much is clear: Immediate further research needs to be done in these areas before we can reach a reasonable conclusion on the safety of these foods. It's worth noting that even a *pro*-biotechnology scientific panel of the National Academy of Sciences in the U.S. admitted in an April 2000 study that more caution and more safety testing are necessary before Americans can be reassured that gene-altered foods are safe.

3

WHAT ARE THE ENVIRONMENTAL HAZARDS OF GE FOOD?

UNLIKE TOXIC chemical pollution released into the environment, which can dissipate over time, genetically engineered crops and animals are living organisms. Genetic pollution is irreversible. It cannot be recalled as it makes its way through our global ecosystem. In this chapter we will look at some of the environmental risks of GE crops including:

- irreversible genetic pollution and drift
- damage to non-target species, beneficial insects, wildlife, and soil fertility
- creation of genetically engineered "superweeds" and "superpests"

- Frankenfish and other mutant bio-invaders
- creation of new plant viruses
- damage to biological diversity

IRREVERSIBLE GENETIC POLLUTION AND DRIFT

GENETIC POLLUTION or drift occurs when the pollen from a genetically engineered plant or crop is carried by the wind or insects and then pollinates the plants (either the same conventional variety as the GE plant or a closely related wild relative) in adjacent fields or in the surrounding environment. Genetic pollution can also occur when GE seeds comingle with non-GE seeds on the farm, in transit, and in seed packaging and distribution facilities.

Once genetically engineered crops are released outside the laboratory, there is no way to prevent them from spreading their altered genes into the environment, nor any way to effectively reverse this process of genetic drift once it's underway. Because they are alive, gene-altered crops are inherently more unpredictable than chemical pollutants—they can reproduce, migrate, and mutate. Wind, rain, birds, bees, and insect pollinators have begun carrying genetically altered pollen and seeds from millions of acres of genetically engineered crops into adjoining fields and non-agricultural lands. This genetic drift has already begun polluting the DNA of crops of organic and non-GE farmers. In addition, the collateral damage from repeated spraying of powerful broad spectrum herbicides such as glyphosate on herbicide resistant crops kills non-target plants and wildlife. Among a growing number of scientific studies documenting genetic drift, pollution, and damage to plant biodiversity and wildlife are the following:

- In 1994, European scientists reported in *Science* magazine that genetically engineered rapeseed or canola plants were spreading herbicide-resistant genes into nearby fields of mustard plants, a wild relative of the rapeseed.[1]

- The British journal *New Scientist* reported on April 17, 1999, that up to 7 percent of non-genetically engineered rapeseed plants in a lab test plot were experiencing genetic contamination from GE rapeseed plants being grown 400 yards away.
- A 1999 study by the Soil Association, the U.K. organization of organic farmers, found that bees were transporting the pollen of GE rapeseed plants more than three miles.
- A 2003 report sponsored by the U.K. government found that pollen from GE canola (rapeseed) can travel up to 16 miles, and recommended that GE canola and sugar beets not be grown in Great Britain because of the threats to wildlife and biodiversity.[2]
- A January 2004 report by the National Academy of Sciences concluded that there don't appear to be any effective ways to prevent genetically engineered material from escaping into the wild.[3]
- A 2004 study in the U.S., carried out by the Union of Concerned Scientists, found that DNA from genetically engineered corn, soybeans, and canola was contaminating non-GE varieties of these crops.[4]
- Other studies have shown that genetically engineered radishes, sorghum, and sunflowers can easily transfer their altered DNA to wild relatives.

GENETIC POLLUTION THREATENS BOTH ORGANIC AND CONVENTIONAL FARMERS

ORGANIC FARMERS and conventional farmers trying to grow certified non-GE crops are up in arms about genetic pollution. If your crop "tests positive" for the presence of genetically engineered organisms, you can't sell it as organic or GE-free, which means that you may not be able to sell your crop at all, or at best you'll get a lower price for it. And you may find that your crop next year is contaminated as well. In 1998 corn grown on an organic farm in Texas was contaminated with genetic drift from GE corn on a nearby farm, causing an entire wholesale shipment of organic corn chips worth several hundred thousand dollars to be destroyed by authorities in Europe.

A number of organic growers in the United States have found their corn and other crops were testing positive for the presence of genetically modified organisms, even though they didn't plant genetically engineered seeds. Seeing that there is no way to avoid at least a certain degree of genetic drift and pollution, European regulators have begun the process of setting an "allowable limit" for genetic contamination of certified organic and certified non-GE foods. American organic certification bodies have initiated a similar discussion.

In Britain, the government is telling organic farmers that they are just going to have to accept some level of genetic contamination. "We cannot have 100 percent total purity because we do not have the appropriate barriers," the British Food Safety Minister told organic groups. "The organic movement has to recognize and find a way of living with contamination from other crops."[5]

In a survey released in 2003, the public interest group Organic Farming Research Foundation found that 11 percent of U.S. organic farmers had already detected GMO contamination in their fields, mainly in corn crops. According to OFRF President Ron Rosmann, a diversified organic farmer from Harlan, Iowa, "This new data supports OFRF's call for a moratorium on the release of GMOs until there is a solid regulatory framework that prevents genetic pollution and assigns liability for the damages imposed by GMO contamination."[6]

Of course, setting allowable residue limits for GE contamination will not solve the problem. The basic fact is this: Once genetic pollution begins, it is virtually impossible to stop. It will inevitably spread and biologically accumulate in the environment over time. For this reason there is a growing demand among farmers and environmentalists for a global moratorium on all GE crops. In December 1999 a global class-action lawsuit by organic, as well as conventional farmers and consumer organizations was filed against several biotech companies, citing genetic drift and economic harm to farmers as one of its primary allegations.

In 2002, a thousand organic farmers in Canada filed a multi-million dollar lawsuit against biotech companies Aventis (now owned by Bayer) and Monsanto, claiming that the planting of millions of acres of GE rapeseed in Canada had polluted the countryside and their crops, making it all but impossible to grow non-GE or organic canola. The organic farmers also pointed out that the future commercialization of Monsanto's GE herbicide-resistant wheat, under consideration for approval by Canadian and U.S. regulatory agencies, would result in further pollution and crop contamination.[7]

BT-RESISTANT SUPERPESTS: A CRISIS FOR ORGANIC AGRICULTURE

BT, THE universally used abbreviation for *Bacillus thuringiensis,* is a natural biopesticide that derives from a soil bacterium that naturally repels certain plant pests such as potato beetles, corn borers, and cotton bollworms. Natural forms of Bt have been utilized by organic and low-chemical input farmers for decades (usually as a spray) on crops such as tomatoes, potatoes, corn, and cotton. Since Bt in spray form degrades in sunlight and evaporates from plant surfaces within a short period of time (roughly seventy-two hours), farmers don't have to worry about Bt residues contaminating the food crop or toxic Bt residues building up in the soil.

As with all natural biopesticides, organic farmers use Bt spray only when absolutely necessary, and they use only the smallest amounts possible to ward off pest attacks that threaten their crops. Organic farmers know that if they overuse an emergency biopesticide such as Bt, pests will inevitably develop resistance to the spray, and then they will have nothing, short of toxic pesticides—which are prohibited on organic farms—to save their crops. Non-GE Bt sprays are the most important emergency pest control agent for organic and low-chemical use farmers in the world.

Unfortunately, Bt has been the victim of its own long-term success rate. Several companies have genetically engineered a variety of crops by splicing Bt into the plant itself. Corn, cotton, and potatoes have all been genetically engineered with Bt. However, genetically engineered Bt crops differ completely from organic or conventional crops that have merely been sprayed with a Bt spray:

- GE Bt-spliced plants are designed to continually manufacture the Bt toxin or poison in every cell of their organism.
- GE crops produce Bt toxin that is 10–50 times more powerful than traditional Bt crop sprays.
- The Bt toxin in GE plants does not readily decompose.
- Genetically engineered Bt remains as residue on the food crop.
- Some scientists have warned that certain GE Bt formulations may set off food allergies.
- Gene-altered Bt builds up in the soil when it leaches through the plant's root system, as well as when the plant's leaves fall on the ground and when the entire post-harvest plant is plowed back into the soil.

Because gene-altered Bt plants constantly pump out high-potency levels of Bt, lab and field tests indicate that common plant pests such as cotton bollworms, budworms, corn borers, and potato beetles, living under constant pressure from GE crops, will likely soon evolve into "superpests" completely immune to Bt biopesticide sprays. This will present a serious danger for organic and sustainable farmers whose biological pest management practices will be unable to cope with increasing numbers of superpests.

A 1999 article in *Science* magazine (284: 965–67) pointed out that European corn borers resistant to the Bt toxin may carry this resistance as a dominant, rather than a recessive trait, with the consequence that these Bt superpests will likely breed and multiply at a much faster rate than previously expected. This in turn could quickly render non-GE Bt pesticidal sprays ineffective. A related study at the University of Arizona on the pink bollworm, a major cotton pest, found that Bt-resistant bollworms reach sexual maturity faster than regular bollworms, thus assuring they will mate with each other, rather than non-resistant bollworms. This, in turn, will speed up the process at which Bt-resistant bollworms will breed and proliferate.

ORGANIC FARMERS SUE THE EPA

REACTING TO the dangers of crop pests developing resistance to Bt, in February of 1999, the International Federation of Organic Agriculture Movements, Greenpeace, the Center for Food Safety, and twenty-eight other public interest groups filed a federal lawsuit against the U.S. government to have all genetically engineered Bt crops pulled off the market. Commenting on the lawsuit, Benedikt Haerlin, Greenpeace International's coordinator of genetic engineering campaigning, stated: "The approval of Bt plants is a classic example of how destructive agricultural practices are now being extended from chemical to biological warfare against nature."

Jim Gerritsen, a Maine organic farmer and one of the plaintiffs in the Bt lawsuit, stated, "We consider the transgenic application of Bt to be unwise because of the high likelihood that they will rapidly accelerate resistance to Bt. Should we ever lose Bt, our ability as natural farmers to grow quality produce will be in serious question."[7] Gerritsen and others have pointed out that non-genetically engineered, natural strains of Bt have been used as a biological pesticide for decades to protect crops and forests without harmful effects on the environment or human health. Natural Bt sprays are the single most important bio-pesticide in the world—with annual sales of over $60 million in the U.S. alone, according to the Center for Food Safety.

In 2001, after federal courts failed to ban GE corn spliced with Bt, the U.S. Enviornmental Protection Agency renewed the license for biotech companies to cultivate Bt corn and other crops for an additional 7 years.

MONARCH BUTTERFLIES
ARE GROUNDED BY GE

IN THE most dramatic and widely publicized GE story of 1999, *Nature* magazine published a letter from Cornell University scientists in its May 20 issue indicating that pollen from genetically engineered Bt corn crops is poisonous to Monarch butterflies. The scientists found that 44 percent of Monarch caterpillars that ate milkweed leaves (their exclusive food source) dusted with the pollen of Bt corn died. Those that survived suffered from a 60 percent weight loss. The Cornell researchers warned that their test results "have potentially profound implications for the conservation of Monarch butterflies" and that more research on the environmental risks of genetically engineered crops are required.

Headline stories of the threat to what the press dubbed "the Bambi of the insect world" brought home the fact that millions of acres of GE crops are under cultivation in the U.S., with untold damage already being done to the environment and living creatures. Although Monsanto and the biotech industry immediately tried to undercut the Monarch story, complaining that the studies were carried out in a laboratory rather than in the fields, findings by scientists from Iowa State University conducted in and around fields planted with Bt corn showed a 19 percent mortality rate within 48 hours for Monarch butterflies that feasted on milkweed with the levels of Bt pollen.[8]

In an August 11, 1999, petition sent to the Environmental Protection Agency by the Union of Concerned Scientists and leading environmental organizations, the groups warned that it is not only Monarch butterflies that are at risk from poisoning by Bt crops:

"EPA failed to assess risks of toxic pollen to non-target Lepidoptera [Monarchs]. . . . Of special concern is the failure to evaluate impacts on the 18 moths and butterflies listed as threatened under the federal Endangered Species Act."

Responding to the Monarch controversy, then USDA head Dan Glickman emphasized in interviews that "We can't force-feed consumers. . . . There are certainly more and more questions being asked about biotechnology, and those questions must be answered." European Union and Japanese authorities reacted to the Monarch study by announcing that previous approvals for Bt crops in Europe and Japan will now have to be reviewed and possibly reversed. Greenpeace threatened a lawsuit unless the prior EU approvals for several Bt crops were canceled. The Bt-Monarch controversy comes on the heels of other recent studies showing that:

- Bt-spliced crops kill beneficial insects such as lacewings and ladybugs.
- Bt-spliced crops kill beneficial soil microorganisms.
- Bt-spliced crops damage soil fertility, and may be harming insect-eating birds.

At an international meeting of entomologists (scientists who study insects) in Basel, Switzerland, in March 1999, experts warned that genetically engineered Bt crops are exuding 10–20 times the amount of toxins contained in conventional (non-GE) Bt sprays, are harming beneficial insects and soil microorganisms, and may likely be harming insect-eating bird populations. The scientists called for a moratorium on commercial planting of Bt crops.

COSTS TO BENEFICIAL INSECTS, BIRDS, AND BEES?

MANY FARMERS rely on beneficial insects, birds, and bees to ward off pests and keep their farms healthy. What effect GE crops will have on these "farm helpers" is unclear. Among other recent studies on the damage of GE crops to beneficial insects, Swiss research published in the journal *Environmental Entomology* in April 1998 indicates that the mortality rate of the green lacewing, a beneficial insect, rose 150 percent after they ingested corn borers, a leading corn pest, which had eaten Bt corn. Meanwhile *Consumer Reports* (September 1999) summarized EU research, indicating that bees fed proteins from genetically engineered rapeseed plants "had trouble learning to distinguish between the smells of flowers" and suffered increased mortality rates. In October 2003, a British government study found that GE crops significantly reduced the biodiversity of fields, including lowering the populations of beetles, butterflies, bees, and other insects.[9] In Britain, English Nature, the government's official wildlife advisory committee, called for a moratorium on the planting of GE crops, citing likely damage to birds and other wildlife.

BELOW THE SURFACE—SOIL DAMAGE

A CRITICAL element to the success of farming is healthy soil. Genetically engineered Bt pollen clearly poses some dangers by traveling through the air, but what is happening in the soil could be just as significant.

The Fall/Winter 1998 issue of the Union of Concerned Scientists' *Gene Exchange* reported on research showing that genetically engineered Bt crops are building up Bt toxins in the soil, thereby damaging the soil food web and beneficial soil microorganisms. A study cited in *Soil Biology and Biochemistry* showed that engineered Bt does not break down in soils as readily as conventional Bt sprays, and likely remains after crop harvest in the soil or in compost.[10]

In yet another disturbing study, New York University researchers revealed in the December 2, 1999, issue of *Nature* that Bt toxins from genetically engineered crops are leaching into the soil through the plants' root systems, damaging or killing beneficial soil microorganisms, and disrupting the soil food web. The report also documents that Bt toxins bind with soil particles for up to 243 days and remain toxic to soil insects for long periods of time.[11]

Researchers have found three known methods by which genetically engineered Bt toxins are reaching the soil:

1. farmers' plowing under plant debris after harvest;
2. pollen from genetically engineered crops falling to the ground;
3. engineered Bt exudating through the roots of the plant.

This research underlines the urgent need for more study into what GE crops are doing to living organisms below the soil.

DEADLY GE SOIL MICROORGANISMS

IT'S NOT only Bt crops that threaten soil ecology. At the annual meeting of the Ecological Society of America in 1994, Dr. Elaine Ingham and other scientists from Oregon State University reported that a genetically engineered soil bacterium, Klebsiella planticola, developed by a European genetic engineering company to produce ethanol alcohol from crop wastes, completely destroyed the root systems of plants which were subsequently planted in the gene-altered soil. Dr. Ingham warned that if the GE Klebsiella planticola bacteria had been commercialized, an irreversible ecological disaster would have taken place whereby vast expanses of farmland would have been rendered infertile forever.[12] Following the study the biotech company holding the patent on the GE Klebsiella withdrew its plans for commercialization.

Environmental Protection Agency whistle-blowers issued similar, if slightly less alarming, warnings in 1997 protesting government approval of a GE soil bacterium called Rhizobium melitoli, designed to increase nitrogen fixation in the soil. Despite these warnings, commercialization of the Rhizobium microorganism has gone forward.

THE LARGEST sector of genetically engineered crops are those designed to be herbicide-resistant. Yet, these crops pose some of the most significant threats to farms. There is already evidence that weeds like wild mustard, wild radish, ryegrass, or goat grass are developing resistance to herbicides because of overexposure. As a result, in the future these new "superweeds" will require stronger, more toxic chemicals to control them.

Farmers and scientists have known for decades that overuse of a particular pesticide or herbicide tends to make weeds or insect pests resistant or immune to that particular pesticide. Now scientists warn us that genetically engineering major agricultural crops to be herbicide-resistant threatens to make the problem of weed and pest-resistance even worse. Since herbicide-resistant GE crops' main characteristic is their ability to survive megadoses of broad-spectrum herbicides, weeds will inevitably develop resistance to commonly used herbicides such as glyphosate, glufosinate, and bromoxynil. Even the genetic engineering companies admit resistance will occur. In fact after only a few years of commercialization we are already seeing the emergence of the first "superweeds" in Europe as GE rapeseed (canola) spreads its herbicide-resistance traits to related weeds such as wild mustard plants.[13] And in Canada, scientists reported in February 2000 that weeds near genetically engineered canola had developed resistance to three different herbicides, making the so-called "superweed" an unfortunate reality.[14] In recent years, farmers from California to Mississippi to Maryland have reported Roundup-resistant ryegrass and horseweed.

THE ONE THAT GOT AWAY—FRANKENFISH

THE GENETIC engineering of fish such as carp, salmon, and trout to grow larger poses serious potential environmental risks.

Scientists have already engineered trout to grow almost eight times larger than normal-size trout. A/F Protein, a Massachusetts-based company, is gearing up for large-scale production of engineered trout and Atlantic salmon hoping to get approval from the U.S. government to put these products on the market. Worldwide, researchers have found the genetic keys to rapid growth in at least eleven commercially valuable fish species, including shrimp growing at the University of Connecticut.[15]

What will happen to wild fish and marine species when scientists release into the environment fish that are twice as large, and eat twice as much food, as their wild counterparts? A number of studies have already shown that (non-GE) non-native commercial breeds of Atlantic salmon escaping from fish farms on the west coast have spread diseases that have devastated native Pacific wild salmon. Researchers at Purdue University concluded that just a small number of growth-enhanced GE fish could eradicate large populations of wild fish. Larger GE fish attract more mates and quickly spread their characteristics throughout the population. However, the offspring of these fish have reduced reproductive capability and so reduce the health of the entire population.[16]

Problems associated with the genetic engineering process of fish have already convinced one previously interested company to back away from the technology. New Zealand–based King Salmon Co. Ltd. announced that it would bury the remains of genetically engineered salmon it had produced that ended up with deformed heads and other abnormalities.[17]

IDENTICAL TREES

FOREST GROUPS are already concerned about the effects genetically engineered trees might have on fragile ecosystems. These trees are designed to grow faster and more uniformly, and to resist pests and herbicides. A December 1999 report by the World Wildlife Fund (WWF) found that a large number of genetically engineered trees are already being planted around the world without proper safety measures. The report warns that commercial production of genetically engineered trees could begin soon in Chile, China, and Indonesia. According to the WWF report, the threat of genetic pollution is high. Other threats to the environment include possible new superweeds. There could also be unintended impacts on non-target species when trees are engineered for pest resistance and herbicide tolerance.

CREATION OF NEW PLANT VIRUSES

ANOTHER TYPE of genetically engineered crop is one that is gene-spliced so as to be resistant to viruses. Unfortunately, virus-spliced crops pose a whole new set of problems. To the average consumer, plant viruses may seem rather esoteric, but in fact they are extremely important to our food supply. On the one hand plant viruses, especially in a period of accelerated climate change, can devastate our food crops or greatly reduce yields. On the other hand, certain plant viruses are beneficial in that they keep other undesirable weeds and food crop pests in check. Of course the more out of balance things get on agricultural land, the more weeds there are, and at least on a non-organic farm, the more herbicides get sprayed—ending up as toxic residues in the ground water and on our food crops.

Research by plant virologists indicates that gene-splicing may result in unanticipated outcomes and dangerous surprises that could damage important food crops and reduce biodiversity. Dr. Gus de Zoeten and Dr. Richard Allison, well-respected experts on plant pathology, after conducting experiments at Michigan State University in 1994, found that gene-splicing plants with viruses (to produce virus-resistant GE crops such as the yellow crookneck squash) can cause plant viruses to mutate into new, more virulent forms at a rate considerably higher than that theorized by the biotech industry or U.S. regulatory agencies.[18] New virulent plant viruses in the environment could potentially cause catastrophic crop losses and kill off important plant species. Since virus-spliced transgenic varieties of plants continually express the viral gene in all of their cells, the probability of recombining with other plant viruses is greatly increased.

On November 3, 1999, the *New York Times* reported that the USDA approved several applications for commercialization of virus-spliced squash by Asgrow Seeds (a division of Monsanto) with little or no scientific data supporting industry claims that "wild squash was unlikely to interbreed with genetically engineered squash." The USDA made this ruling despite considerable worry among plant virologists that this type of gene-splicing could produce new superweeds that would be immune to the common plant viruses in the environment that keep these weeds in check. In other words, virus-resistant superweeds could evolve would overrun and devastate crop lands and the surrounding environment.

GE CROPS PROMOTE
DEADLY PLANT FUNGUS

TWO ARTICLES published in 2003 indicate that GE herbicide-resistant wheat and soybeans sprayed with glyphosate give rise to a damaging plant fungus called Fusarium. In several studies, researchers found that repeated spraying with glyphosate on GE Roundup Ready soybeans increased plant pathogens in the soil, namely Fusarium fungus, leading to "Sudden Death Syndrome" in the plants.[19] Other studies, sponsored by the Canadian government, indicated that repeated spraying of Roundup herbicide on GE wheat plants led to an increased incidence of Fusarium "head blight," a toxin that makes the wheat unfit for human or animal consumption.[20]

IN ADDITION to environmental damage, perhaps even more alarming to consumers are reports from Iowa, published in 2002, that pigs fed a steady diet of Bt corn seem to have developed reproductive problems, making them unable to become pregnant. Iowa pig farmer Jerry Rosman, as well as a number of his neighbors, told the press that sows fed exclusively on Bt corn developed symptoms of "false pregnancy," swelling up but remaining infertile. Once one of the farmers stopped feeding their pigs Bt corn, they were able to get pregnant and give birth.Laboratory tests revealed the Iowa pig farmers' corn contained high levels of Fusarium mold. Rosman says researchers tracked the Fusarium down to four strains, and two of them (Fusarium subglutinans and Fusarium monlliforme) were consistent in all the producers' samples.[21]

Evidence that genetically engineered crops are harming the environment is rapidly accumulating. The long-term effects of this new technology on the soil, other insects, and farm animals—key components of a farmer's ecosystem—are still virtually unknown. But the number of red flags appears to be increasing by the month.

4

WHAT ARE THE SOCIAL AND ETHICAL HAZARDS OF GENETICALLY ENGINEERED FOODS AND CROPS?

THE IMPACT of genetically engineered foods and crops extends well beyond the environment and human health. GE foods and crops are changing the face of U.S. and global agriculture and posing troublesome socioeconomic and ethical questions, questions that fall into the following categories:

- The social and economic hazards of GE: the escalation and exacerbation of negative trends already manifest in the globalization and industrialization of agriculture.
- The political hazards of GE: the threats to national food security, both at home and abroad, the potential dislocation of hundreds of millions of small farmers and rural villagers, and the magnification of monopoly trends already evident in industrial agriculture.

- The ethical hazards of GE: the "slippery slope" of patenting and owning living life forms.
- The threat that patents on seeds, so-called intellectual property rights, will prevent the majority of the world's farmers from saving and exchanging seeds, as they have done for millennia.
- The genetic theft or biopiracy of the biological resources and genetic biodiversity found in nature and particularly in the developing world.

THE HEALTH OF THE FARM

FOR OVER 10,000 years farmers have been saving and selecting the seeds of their "best" agricultural food crops and herbs. If a plant variety was easy to harvest; produced a good yield; tasted good; did well in a particular type of soil, exhibited vigor or hardiness to survive pests, diseases, and a variety of weather and climate changes or stresses; then farmers have saved these seeds, exchanged them with their neighbors, and planted them for the next harvest. By planting a variety of naturally pollinating seeds, each with their own slightly different characteristics, farmers were able to raise resilient crops with genetic variance that allowed them to be brought to harvest. Without the work of these seed savers and diligent horticulturists over many centuries, we as consumers would not be able to enjoy the variety, quantity, and quality of the foods we eat and take for granted today.

Over time, thousands of different varieties of rice, wheat, corn, potatoes, and hundreds of other food and fiber crops were developed and nurtured, guaranteeing that just about every ecosystem and every microclimate in the world had an ample supply and diversity of seeds and plant species to survive. Farmers and ranchers of course did the same thing with their domesticated farm animals, selecting and breeding the "best" animals for the world's varying climates and terrain. Until recently, the typical farmer in the United States and around the world cultivated a variety of field crops as well as garden vegetables, and also raised animals, who provided not only meat, milk, and eggs, but wool, leather, and manure for fertilizer.

The need for plant diversity became evident in Ireland in 1845 when a million people starved to death because a potato blight devastated the entire monoculture (single variety) potato crop planted on the island. A similar disaster occurred in the U.S. in 1970 when a corn disease or blight ravaged the national corn harvest, destroying 15 percent of the entire crop and reducing yields by as much as 50 percent.

INDUSTRIAL AGRICULTURE:
THE DEATH OF DIVERSITY

WITH THE onset of modern agriculture this approach to farming began to change. Over the past century agriculture has become more industrialized and specialized with a vast decrease in the varieties of individual crops being grown. Agribusiness seed corporations learned to mass-produce "hybrid" seeds by crossing or interbreeding different purebred strains of particularly high-yielding or disease-resistant plants. Whereas farmers had traditionally cross-bred a wide variety of plants (and animals) on a small scale for their own use and to trade or exchange in their local communities, new giant seed companies such as Pioneer Hi-Bred rose up to sell their hybrid seeds to thousands and eventually millions of farmers.

The advantage of hybrid seeds is that you get a higher yield, producing more of a particular crop per acre. As market forces and the consolidation of agriculture companies pushed modern farmers from polyculture (multiple crops) to monoculture (one crop), from variety to volume, farmers abandoned traditional self-pollinating (non-hybrid) varieties of seeds and began purchasing hybrid seeds and concentrating on producing vast quantities of one or two cash crops such as corn, sorghum, wheat, and cotton.

The economic disadvantage of hybrid seeds is that farmers need to buy a lot more chemical fertilizers, pesticides, and irrigation equipment, which not only raise their costs and make them dependent on bank loans or government credit, but also negatively impact the soil and the environment. And in many cases, banks have made credit dependent on whether farmers are using the most updated technology. Another fundamental problem with hybrid seeds is that the plants they produce are generally sterile or do not "breed true." If you tried saving your seeds after harvest, either you'd get no crop, a reduced crop, or a crop with lower yields and different characteristics than those in the original hybrid strain. Many farmers stopped saving and exchanging seeds and instead went back to the seed dealers every year for their supply of ever more expensive seeds. The result has been a dramatic decline in plant and crop varieties and a dangerous overreliance on a handful of vulnerable hybrid seed types.

As Michael Fox states in his book *Eating with Conscience: The Bioethics of Food*:

> Conservationists estimate that we have lost more than half the varieties of the world's 20 most important food crops that existed at the beginning of the century. These include corn, rice, wheat, potatoes, and bananas. Over the same period we have allowed 80 percent of the varieties of horticultural fruit crops in the United States to disappear. More than one-third of livestock and poultry breeds in the United States are rare or in decline, and half of the breeds in Europe that existed at the turn of the century are now extinct.[1]

GE—FATAL TO AGRICULTURAL DIVERSITY?

FURTHER LIMITING farmers' choices, genetic engineering companies have begun to steadily buy up major seed companies around the world. As a January 7, 2000, study by the Research Advancement Foundation International (RAFI) points out, a powerful complex of five transnational Life Science corporations (Monsanto, Aventis, Novartis, Dupont, and Dow) now control "68 percent of the global agrochemical market and over 20 percent of the commercial seed trade worldwide."[2] It is estimated that as a result of a series of acquisitions and mergers, DuPont and Monsanto together now own 73 percent of corn seed produced in the U.S.

AGBIOTECH'S FIVE JUMBO GENE GIANTS

Company Global Rankings by Sector (in U.S. $millions—based on 1998 revenues)

Aventis = Hoechst + Rhone Poulenc (France)

    Agrochemical Ranking: #2—$4,675

    Seed Ranking: not ranked—$134

Monsanto (USA) + Pharmacia & UPjohn

    Agrochemical Ranking: #3—$4,030

    Seed Ranking: #2—$1,800

Dupont (USA) = Pioneer Hybrid

    Agrochemical Ranking: #4—$3,155

    Seed Ranking: #1—$1,835

Syngenta = Novartis + AstraZeneca

    Agrochemical Ranking: #1—$7,050

    Seed Ranking: #3—$1,000

    #4—AstraZeneca—$12,750

    #7—Novartis—$11,175

Dow Chemical (USA)

    Agrochemical Ranking: #7—$2,130

    Seed Ranking: not ranked—$162 million

        Sources: Information based on RAFI research, AGROW agrochemical rankings and SCRIP Pharmaceutical League Table, December, 1999.

These new biotech seed conglomerates have a simple marketing goal—to sell a very limited variety of patented genetically engineered seeds to as many farmers as possible all over the world, just as they have done in the U.S. As Martin Teitel and Kimberly

Wilson put it in their book, *Changing the Nature of Nature*, this phenomena will undoubtedly lead to a qualitative escalation of "genetic erosion" and an ever more serious weakening of plants' resistance to disease, pests, and climate change:

> Plant species in the wild are less vulnerable to insects and diseases because they have a broader genetic base to work from. While such genetic erosion is irreversible, we must guard against a further loss of biodiversity—the diversity genetic engineering threatens most. When insects and microbes ravage monocultures of [genetically engineered] food, genetic engineers become 'treadmill plant breeders,' continually forced to develop new pest-resistant varieties that survive for a while— until the pests adapt to that variety.[3]

OPENING PANDORA'S BOX

READ ANY farming magazine and it's hard to miss. Page after page of relentless advertisements for the latest genetically engineered crops. For a struggling farmer, this technology, touted as the future of agriculture, can be tempting. But taking the plunge into genetically engineered crops is not as simple as ordering the seeds. Not only do these new crops bring a new biology to farming, they represent an equally profound shift away from some fundamental rights of farmers. In fact, farmers have been caught in the middle from the beginning, receiving conflicting information on this new technology from seed companies, government regulatory agencies, and food companies.

CONTRACT FARMING

WHEN FARMERS decide to use genetically engineered seeds, they must sign a contract with the seed company that produces them. Farmers do not buy seeds in the traditional sense. Instead, they lease proprietary technology from the seed company. And what they do with that technology is firmly regimented. For one, the contract that farmers are required to sign governs the use of the seeds, and usually includes strict rules that forbid the saving of seeds—the farmer must plant them all that season, and cannot save some for next year. Additionally, the farmer must allow the seed company access to their land at all times. This last provision is the reason why many farmers are still resisting genetically engineered crops—they simply don't want to give up the rights to their land. If provisions of the contract are broken, the farmer is subject to major penalties, and can be sued and seriously fined. These contracts are taken seriously by biotech companies and are enforced to the letter. Monsanto has even employed the feared Pinkerton security firm to enforce its contracts. By the year 2000, Monsanto had already sued 475 farmers for the "crime" of saving or planting their genetically engineered seeds without paying them a royalty payment.[4]

UNCERTAIN MARKETS

WHILE BIOTECH companies are telling farmers they can't survive without genetically engineered crops, the markets tell a different story. According to the American Corn Growers Association (ACGA), in marketing year 1997–98, corn exports to Europe stood at 2 million tons. In marketing year 1998–99, those same exports dropped to 137,000 tons. Soybeans dropped from 11 million tons in 1998 to 6 million tons in 1999. According to the ACGA, American farmers lost at least $814 million in corn sales to Europe between 1998–2003 and even more on soybeans. Between 2000 and 2002, Brazil's share of the world soybean market rose from 24 percent to 30 percent, while the U.S. slice declined from 57 percent to 46 percent.[5] Since 1999 farmers have been getting different signals from the grain wholesalers who actually buy the crops. A. E. Staley, the nation's second largest corn processor, stated in 1999 that they will not accept non-European Union approved genetically engineered corn, while Archer Daniels Midland (ADM) told farmers that they should separate their crops to be sold to foreign markets. Also in 1999 ADM began paying farmers a premium price for non-genetically engineered crops.[6] But a few months later, and in subsequent statements, ADM has declared its support for biotech, sending mixed signals to farmers: "And since improved hybrids will mean more food and better food, it's clear that the mission of biotechnology fits in perfectly with our own. Technology is a major asset in the fight against hunger. ADM will always use it to the greatest advantage."

In 1999 Illinois Cereal Mills, owned by Cargill Inc., began increasing its contracts for crops that aren't genetically engineered. But Cargill itself actively supports genetically engineered crops and accepts GE crops to be processed. Since 1999 both ADM and Cargill have continued hedging their bets, saying they support biotech on the one hand, while nonetheless sourcing and supplying ever-increasing amounts of non-GMO grains to large buyers in Europe and Japan—and putting farmers in a difficult position in the meantime.

U.S. FOOD COMPANIES ARE STARTING TO CHANGE THEIR TUNE

MANY U.S. farmers have felt comfortable with the potential markets for this technology as long as they have seen a united front from the food industry fully supporting biotech crops. The Grocery Manufacturers of America and the National Food Processors Association, among others, have actively supported genetic engineering both in the press and in Washington, D.C. But over the past four years, some major companies began breaking ranks. In February 2000, when Frito-Lay required its contract farmers not to grow genetically engineered corn, it sent shockwaves through the farming community. Infant formula manufacturer Mead Johnson told the press in March 2000 that they intended to "reduce or eliminate" GE ingredients for their infant formula, Enfamil. And perhaps an even more troubling move to farmers was the decision by baby food company Gerber, which is owned by biotech seed producer Novartis, to take genetically engineered food ingredients out of its baby food and go organic in late 1999. In 2002 General Mills warned Monsanto and the biotech industry not to go forward on commercializing genetically engineered wheat, while Anheuser-Busch, Coors, and other major beer companies issued similar warnings regarding GE rice. (More information on companies going GE-free is in chapter 7). Several other major food companies, including Hershey's and McDonald's, have admitted they are taking steps to go GE-free if American consumers demand it. When you throw in the organic and natural food industry—all actively working to source GE-free crops—the united front in the U.S. food industry that originally gave farmers confidence is slowly breaking apart. This is one of the main reasons why GE crop acreage in the U.S. has slowed considerably over the past three years, after explosive growth between 1996 and 2001.

U.S. REGULATORY AGENCIES

U.S. GOVERNMENT regulatory agencies are also wavering. After a decade of telling the public, and farmers, that genetically engineered crops are 100 percent safe, the FDA has made some previously voluntary requirements mandatory because of apparent weaknesses. The EPA announced in early 2000 new requirements for farmers to guard against environmental concerns. These new rules require farmers to set aside 20 to 50 percent of their land to guard against increased pest resistance that is being caused by the biotech seeds. (See chapter 3 for more on this.) The EPA rules place a major burden on farmers to essentially protect the effectiveness of a technology they don't own, by sacrificing part of their farmland. And in April 2000 a panel of the prestigious National Academy of Sciences (NAS) called for more rigorous testing and regulation of GE crops by U.S. regulatory agencies. Early in 2004, a research panel of the NAS concluded that "bioconfinement" of GMO crops in the open environment is virtually impossible.[7]

U.S. FARMERS GET SHORT END ON COST AND SEED SAVING

A PARTICULARLY harsh blow dealt to farmers who have grown genetically engineered soybeans came in a February 2000 U.S. Government General Accounting Office (GAO) report, which reported that Argentine farmers were buying Monsanto's Roundup Ready Soybeans at between $12–$15 per 50-pound bag, while American farmers were paying between $20–$23 for the same bag of seed.[8] Monsanto claims the differential can be explained by differing patent protection in the two countries. Specifically Argentina is not giving Monsanto patent protection on their product. An outraged American Soybean Association, which has been pro-biotech, demanded that Monsanto refund U.S. farmers the difference in price—an offer Monsanto refused. Ironically, the American Soybean Association had lobbied for strong U.S. patent laws—the same patent laws that are now hurting U.S. farmers in comparison to Argentine farmers. In 2004 Monsanto announced that they were suspending sales of GE soybean seeds in Argentina. The company admitted that widespread seed saving and reselling of Roundup Ready soybeans by Argentine farmers, a practice prohibited in the United States, had made their business there unprofitable.[9]

AT RISK WITHOUT A SAFETY NET

ALL FARMERS growing genetically engineered crops face the growing possibility that they will be sued if genetic drift causes pollen from GMO crops or "volunteer" plants that survive harvest to move from their fields onto a neighbor's land. No insurance companies will currently insure genetically engineered crops for genetic pollution. "Genetically modified foods are among the riskiest of all possible insurance exposures that we have today," said Robert Hartwig, the chief economist for the Insurance Information Institute, an industry trade association in New York. "And there's a good reason. No one company knows where this path of genetically modified foods is ultimately going to take us in terms of either human health or environmental contamination."[10]

Representatives from the Biotechnology Industry Organization (the industry's trade group) have said that farmers are responsible for genetic drift that hurts the ability of a neighbor to sell their crop. This has already occurred, as detailed in chapter 3, when an organic corn grower had his crop contaminated with genetically engineered material costing an organic chip maker several hundred thousand dollars. Once again, it is the farmers who stand to bear the costs of the technology's shortcomings, not the seed manufacturers. In response a number of laws have been proposed around the country, and at the federal level, to assign liability to the biotech seed companies in the case of genetic drift. In 2004, in a meeting to implement a global Biosafety Protocol, 87 countries agreed that nations will be held financially liable for GMO exports that damage non-GMO or organic crops in importing countries.

TECHNOLOGY IS COSTING SOME FARMERS

SOME FARMERS have already lost large amounts of money from using genetically engineered crops—in some cases because the technology just didn't work. In Missouri, genetically engineered cotton, designed to be resistant to the herbicide glyphosate, had almost 20,000 acres malfunction in the first year. In some cases the plants dropped their cotton boll, and in others glyphosate killed the plants.[11] In Texas, genetically engineered cotton with the Bt pesticides spliced into it completely failed to stop the cotton bollworm (the target pest). And numerous farmers had problems with uneven growth and lower yields.[12] More recently reports from the field have indicated that repeated spraying of Roundup on herbicide-resistant crops appears to have given rise to a serious plant fungus called Fusarium.[13]

Additionally, GMO products are costing farmers more than they thought. According to analysisdone by Dr. Charles Benbrook, genetically modified crops are requiring more herbicides than farmers were initially led to believe, thus driving up weed management costs. Farmers growing Roundup Ready soybeans used two to five times more herbicide, compared to other popular weed management systems. The increased use of Roundup is already resulting in the emergence of several key weed species developing a tolerance to the herbicide, requiring additional applications to control weeds.[14]

As Charles Benbrook pointed out in 1999, the full Roundup Ready system was costing farmers "an amazing $68.77 per acre, about 50 percent more than the cost of [other] seed plus weed management systems in the Midwest in recent years." This trend would likely deliver "significantly lower average returns to growers," Benbrook predicted.[15] In addition, as indicated in chapter 3, there is evidence of a "yield drag" associated with some Roundup Ready crops, meaning that the RR bushel-to-acre ratio is below that of conventional crops. A yield drag quickly translates into a profitability drag.

THE END OF THE BIOTECH BOOM?

WHILE 1996–1999 represented the boom years for agricultural biotechnology in terms of growth in the number of acres in the U.S. and across the world devoted to growing genetically engineered crops, in the years 2000–2004 growth has been much slower. For example, according to industry sources, global GE crop acreage increased over 675 percent in 1997, 255 percent in 1998, and 143 percent in 1999. In comparison, the biotech industry has reported 11–18 percent growth rates in each of the past four years—reflecting both a saturation or near-saturation of the markets of the four countries growing GE crops on a commercial scale, as well as a reaction to the growing global opposition against GMOs.[16]

Despite intense lobbying by the biotech industry and the U.S. government, no additional countries have stepped forward to grow GE crops on anything other than a token scale over the past four years. While farmers in 110 countries are producing increasingly profitable certified organic crops worth at least $25 billion on the world market, only four countries in the world (the U.S., Canada, Argentina, and China) are growing 99 percent of all commercial GE crops, with a total market value of GE seeds of $4.25 billion.

In the United States and Argentina, where a full 90 percent of all GE crops in the world are cultivated, markets are nearly saturated. For example, 90 percent of soybean farmers in Argentina and 81 percent of soybean farmers in the U.S. are already growing GE soy, the most prevalent GE crop in the world, accounting for 62 percent of all GMOs.[17] In addition, 73 percent of all cotton acreage in the U.S. is already GE, as is over 50 percent of Canada and U.S. canola.[18]

Certainly not all farm groups are supporting the biotech boom. Over thirty farm organizations, representing tens of thousands of small family farmers around the country, have come out opposed to genetically engineered crops. The organizations, including The National Family Farm Coalition, American Corn Growers Association, and Farm Aid, came out with a statement calling for an immediate moratorium on the selling of genetically engineered seeds until "an independent and comprehensive assessment of the social, environmental, health and economic impacts of those products is concluded."

THE TOTAL number of farms in the United States has declined from 6.5 million in 1935 to around 2.12 million in 2002. Most of this decline has taken place among family farms. Even the small number of farmers remaining in 2002 exaggerates how many family farms are left, because most are part-time residential or retirement farms.

Farm Type in 1997	Number	Percent of Farm Sales
Low production, residential and retirement	1,300,000	9
Family sized	575,000	30
Very large corporate farms and family proprietorships	161,000	61[13]

The U.S. Bureau of the Census stopped counting "farm residents" in 1993 because there were so few of them left. (In contrast, in 1900, farm residents made up 35 percent of the total population.[20])

Squeezed by the ever lower prices paid to them by giant agribusiness oligopolies for the food they produce, and, on the other hand, forced to pay the continually increased costs of agricultural inputs (pesticides, fertilizers, seeds, equipment, fuel) to giant chemical and biotech companies, American family farmers are being relentlessly driven off the land.

In order to stay on the land, many of our farmers and ranchers are now forced into poorly paid off-farm employment, which currently provides much of the income they have to meet their survival needs. The only economic "winners" in American agriculture today are large corporate farms; semi-monopolistic grain and commodities traders; seed, biotech, and chemical companies; and giant processors, fast-food restaurants, and supermarket chains. For the rest of rural America, the factory farm, chemical-intensive monoculture cash crop model has proved to be an unmitigated disaster.

Genetically engineered crops are driving a wedge between big farms and smaller farms. The *Financial Times* has reported that in the U.S., larger farms are planting the genetically engineered crops, while smaller farms are more likely to be looking for the GE-free premium price.[21]

A DANGEROUS TECHNOLOGY
FOR A DANGEROUS ECONOMY

IN HIS book, *Farmageddon: Food and the Culture of Biotechnology*, Brewster Kneen points out that genetic engineering is just the latest tool in the hands of transnational food giants and chemical companies to maximize their profits while maintaining control over our food chain and those who produce our food and fiber.[22] With cheaper raw materials, transnational food corporations can force their way into any market in the world and put their smaller competitors out of business. With the advent of NAFTA, for instance, Archer Daniels Midland and Cargill were able to dump hundreds of millions of dollars of taxpayer subsidized corn on Mexican markets and drive over a million small indigenous farmers out of business. Gene engineers look forward to the same "success" with their herbicide resistant and Bt-spliced GE seeds helping "more efficient" farmers beat out their inefficient competitors.

Just as chemical fertilizers, toxic pesticides, hybrid seeds, and factory farming were supposed to lead us into the promised land of the Green Revolution after World War Two, today's bioengineers promise to use genetic engineering to feed the world's growing population, solve modern society's food-related health problems, and clean up the mess they've made with chemical-intensive agriculture over the past fifty years.

Even a number of the agrochemical companies now admit that the Green Revolution of chemical-intensive agriculture is not sustainable. Soils are eroding, crop yields in many places are declining, water for irrigation is ever more limited, and drinking water supplies are increasingly contaminated by agricultural runoff. One billion pounds of toxic pesticides and twelve billion pounds of nitrate chemical fertilizers are being applied to America's farmlands every year, devastating our rural environment. Meanwhile weeds and pests damage or eat up the same proportion of our food crops as they did fifty years ago.

THE BIOTECH CENTURY: DRIVING TWO BILLION "INEFFICIENT" FARMERS OFF THE LAND

THE PROMISE of biotech crops, as championed by the industry, is that it will help feed the poor around the world, and will be necessary as our population grows. Unfortunately, the causes and solutions to hunger are political, not related to food production. In fact, we are producing more food per person than at any time in world history, according to Food First, an international hunger organization. And for the first time in history there are as many people overweight, 1.1 billion, as underfed, according to a March 2000 report by the Worldwatch Institute.[23]

But the root causes of hunger around the world will not be solved with a new technology. As Food First's Peter Rossett wrote in an editorial published in the *New York Times*, "The real problems are poverty and inequality. Too many people are too poor to buy the food that is available or lack land on which to grow it themselves."

Genetically engineered crops do nothing to address these two root causes of hunger. In fact, they will likely do more harm than good. The two primary types of genetically engineered crops thus far, Roundup Ready and Bt, both pose potential pitfalls for the 40 percent (2.4 billion) of the world's 6 billion people that are farmers or rural villagers.

Roundup Ready crops, designed so the farmer must buy the seed and pesticide from the same company, at best produce only equal yields to conventional crops, and in some cases yield decreases. While Roundup crops allow farmers to dump as much pesticides as they want, destroying any neighboring plants around the crop, many non-crop plants are used by farmers in smaller countries as other food sources, or feed for animals.

Genetically engineered Bt crops also allow the seed producer to charge farmers for the seed and pest control system in one shot. At the same time, these crops threaten the effectiveness of natural Bt sprays, used by farmers around the world—particularly organic farmers.

Half of the world's farmers rely on saved seeds for their harvest. Yet, as we pointed out earlier, the contracts farmers sign with GE companies forbid them to do this. The biotech industry has even gone so far, with the assistance of the USDA, to develop technology to make seeds sterile after one growing season—the so-called "Terminator" technology. The Terminator technology has been highly criticized around the world, as well as being the source of many protests by farmers.

Third-world farmers are threatened by genetically engineered crops in the same way that U.S. farmers are. In fact, genetically engineered crops are an instrument to expand the failed U.S. farm policy around the world. Specifically, genetically engineered crops are all about monoculture, producing one cash crop to be sold on the open market. They are not about growing a diverse set of crops to feed yourself, neighbors, and local communities. But it is exactly this kind of sustainable farming that is needed for many countries around the world.

The economic and social dynamic created by genetic engineering, the patenting of transgenic plants and food-producing animals, is leading to universal "bioserfdom" in which farmers will lease their plants and animals from biotech conglomerates and pay permanent royalties on seeds and offspring.

WHAT HAS fueled the biotech crop explosion is not a desire to feed the hungry, but rather the ability of the biotech industry to take out monopoly patents on living organisms such as seeds, plants, animals, microorganisms, and even human cell-lines. In fact without being able to guarantee several decades of legal monopoly (patents typically last twenty years) on its gene-spliced "inventions," the biotech industry would never have invested the billions of dollars in research that have launched this agricultural biotech revolution. Following in the wake of an obscure Supreme Court decision in 1980, which basically overturned a 200-year prohibition on patenting living organisms, researchers and investors realized that they could now "own" entire varieties of plants and animals, as long as they "discovered" them (i.e. mapped out their chemical gene sequences) and/or "invented" them (i.e. performed certain genetic or chemical alterations, no matter how slight, on the natural version of these living organisms). These life patents in turn give the patent holder a legally-binding copyright over a seed or animal, enabling them to charge a "technology fee" to farmers who grow these plants or raise these animals, or a "licensing fee" to scientists who want to research these organisms. "Bio-prospectors" have now spread out across the globe, searching for commercially valuable, patentable plants, herbs, insects, micro-organisms, and human cell-lines.

Vandana Shiva, the India-based scientist and critic of biotechnology has noted: "Biodiversity has been redefined as 'biological inventions' to make patenting of life forms less controversial."[24]

The moral and ethical problem of allowing patents on living organisms is basically this: Where do you draw the line? If it's legal to patent a living microorganism, then it's legal to patent a seed or a plant. If you can patent a plant, then the door is wide open for genetically engineering and patenting animals and human cell-lines, or even body parts, or even people. A British woman recently applied for a patent on herself, both to protect herself, but also to prove a point about the excesses of the current patent system. Scientists are already talking about a major new industry transplanting the organs of genetically engineered animals into humans, cloning humans, and improving the "genetic defects" of animals and humans. Unless U.S. patent laws are changed or enforced differently, and we go back to our longstanding tradition of prohibiting patents on living organisms, it is very likely that the slippery slope we are now on will turn into an avalanche—leading us headlong into a Brave New World where nothing is sacred, everything can be genetically engineered, and human eugenics becomes a technical and commercial, rather than an ethical, issue.

Andrew Kimbrell, attorney and bioethicist, summarizes the historic questions and ethical dilemmas posed by genetically engineering and patenting life forms:

> Embarking on the long journey in which corporations and governments eventually become the brokers of the blueprints of life raises some of the most disturbing and important questions ever to face humanity: Do scientists and corporations have the right to alter the genetic code of life forms at will? Should we alter the genetic structure of the entire living kingdom in the name of utility or profit? . . . Is there something sacred about life, or should life forms . . . be viewed simply as commodities in the new bio-tech marketplace? Is the genetic makeup of all living things the common heritage of all, or can it be appropriated by corporations and governments?"[25]

BIOPIRACY: THE NEW GENETIC COLONIALISM

AS WE noted earlier in this chapter, the painstaking seed saving and farming practices of indigenous and traditional peasants over thousands of years, most often carried out by peasant women, are responsible for most of the genetic richness and vitality found in the varieties of seeds and crops that we enjoy today, from corn, wheat, and rice to hundreds of other food (and medicinal) plants and crops. But from the legal standpoint of the biotech and seed industry, the original inventors and custodians of seeds and plants have no rights whatsoever. Under current Life Patent regimes, only licensed patent holders, typically corporations and research laboratories, have "intellectual property rights." Companies need only to "discover" and expropriate traditional seed and plant varieties (most of which are located in the developing world), chemically or genetically alter them somewhat, and then claim them as their proprietary patented varieties. The farmers and communities who developed these seed varieties, some of which have generated billions of dollars in sales and profits for corporations, get nothing. In fact small farmers and indigenous people can and are being sued and prosecuted for intellectual property rights violations, for the "crime" of saving or planting seed varieties that they themselves and their ancestors developed.

As Indian food activist Vandana Shiva points out, life patenting and so-called "bio-prospecting" amount to little more than a modern version of piracy or colonialism, which she calls "biopiracy." As Shiva states: "Through intellectual property rights, an attempt is made to take away what belongs to nature, to farmers and to women, and to term this invasion improvement and progress."[26]

THE TERMINATOR GENE: TERMINATING SMALL FARMERS & BIODIVERSITY

THE HIGHLY controversial "Terminator" technology is perhaps the clearest example we've seen yet of the social and economic hazards of agricultural genetic engineering. The Terminator technology, euphemistically described by its inventors as a "Technology Protection System," uses genetic engineering to make seeds sterile, to eliminate a plant's natural ability to propagate or reproduce itself. This means that farmers who plant Terminator seeds will have no choice but to go back every year to purchase ever more expensive GE seeds and chemical inputs from a handful of global biotech/seed monopolies. Despite warnings from a broad range of public interest and consumer groups worldwide that Terminator seeds could literally destroy the livelihoods of hundreds of millions of small farmers who depend on saving seeds, and who cannot afford to buy high-priced hybrid or GE seeds, proponents of genetic engineering have pushed ahead with research on the Terminator. Likewise warnings from scientists that the genetic drift of Terminator genes into the environment could cause near-by crops and plants to become sterile has fallen on deaf ears.

FROM TERMINATOR TO TRAITOR

SINCE 1998 dozens of other Terminator patents have been filed for in countries all over the world by companies such as Monsanto and Novartis. Global opposition to the Terminator technology, however, grew to such a level in 1999 that Monsanto promised not to commercialize its continuing research. The USDA, Delta and Pine Land Company, and other patent holders, however, have yet to make such a promise. And as the public interest group RAFI (Research Advancement Foundation International) has pointed out, genetic engineering companies are already working on an even more insidious "second generation" Terminator technology, which RAFI has dubbed the "Traitor Technology." This "trait" or Traitor Technology will accomplish the same basic goal of the Terminator Technology by inhibiting the yield, flowering, or repro-duction of GE crops unless they are sprayed or treated with the proprietary chemicals of the Traitor Technology patent holders. This Traitor Technology not only guarantees that farmers will have to return to the seed companies each year, but that their chemical inputs will have a guaranteed market.

THE GENETIC engineering and patenting of animals reduces sentient living creatures to the status of manufactured products and will result in a escalation of the already institutionalized cruelty of industrialized factory farming. In January 1994, the USDA announced that scientists had completed genetic "road maps" for cattle and pigs, a precursor to ever more experimentation on live animals. In addition to the cruelty inherent in such experimentation (the "mistakes" are born with painful deformities, crippled, blind, and so on), these "manufactured" creatures have no greater value to their "creators" than mechanical inventions. Animals genetically engineered for use in laboratories, such as the infamous "Harvard mouse," which contains a human cancer-causing gene that will be passed down to all succeeding generations, were created to suffer. A purely reductionist science, biotechnology reduces all life to bits of information (genetic code) that can be arranged and rearranged at whim. Stripped of their integrity and sacred qualities, animals who are merely objects to their "inventors" will be treated as such. Currently, hundreds of genetically engineered "freak" animals are awaiting patent approval from the federal government. One can only wonder, after the wholesale gene-altering and patenting of animals, will GE "designer babies" be next?

Aside from scientific questions, it is clear that genetically engineered crops represent a sea change in the way we look at agriculture. And if genetically engineered crops become the dominant form of agriculture, they will change the agri-economy forever. The technology also raises uncomfortable ethical and moral questions about tampering with genetic codes. In the end, there appears to be little consideration of the monumental ethical and moral impacts genetic engineering has on the world.

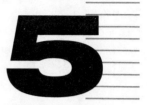

HOW ARE GENETICALLY ENGINEERED FOODS REGULATED IN THE U.S. AND WORLDWIDE?

THERE IS a stark difference between the approach U.S. regulatory agencies take toward genetically engineered foods and the policies of most other industrialized countries. In a nutshell, U.S. agencies treat genetically engineered foods no differently than other foods—requiring neither mandatory safety testing nor labeling. Other nations have followed an approach more consistent with "The Precautionary Principle," which states that when there is scientific uncertainty on the effects of a new technology, the technology must be proven safe before it enters the marketplace.

For example, France placed an immediate moratorium on growing certain types of genetically engineered Bt crops after Cornell University researchers found that pollen from gene-altered corn was toxic to the Monarch butterfly (see chapter 3 for more details). Germany pulled Novartis Bt corn off the market after it determined that antibiotic resistance genes used in the crop could effect the use of antibiotics in that country.

Globally, the United Nation's Food and Agriculture Organization utilized the precautionary principle when it urged caution in March 2000 on GE crops because of unanswered questions about environmental and human health effects. The European Union (EU) has taken the lead in emphasizing precautionary measures when regulating genetically engineered foods and crops. In June 1999, the European Environment Ministers declared a de facto moratorium on the market approval of new genetically engineered foods in Europe until further safety testing has been completed. The EU has not approved a new genetically engineered crop or food since April 1998. And in January 2000, the EU agreed to label all processed foods that contain at least 1 percent of genetically engineered soybean or corn. This policy applies to all fifteen EU member nations. The EU has gone through a long and complicated process and appears to be close to establishing a regulatory system that would allow the approval of some GE crops, with strict labeling and traceability standards.

Before looking at the U.S. regulatory system for genetically engineered foods, you might find it helpful to read about policies and company actions in other countries. The Center for Food Safety and the International Forum on Globalization have compiled a comprehensive list and map of the GE food and crop policies of all the nations in the world. The map is being regularly updated, so check their Web site, www.centerforfoodsafety.org, for the latest details.

COUNTRIES WITH A BAN OR MORATORIUM ON GE FOOD AND CROPS:

- Albania
- Algeria
- Austria

- Belgium
- Benin
- Croatia
- Denmark
- Egypt
- El Salvador
- Finland
- France
- Georgia
- Germany
- Greece
- Ireland
- Italy
- Luxenburg
- The Netherlands
- New Zealand
- Paraguay
- Peru
- Portugal
- Spain
- Sweden
- Thailand
- The United Kingdom

COUNTRIES WITH REQUIRED LABELING OF GE FOODS AND CROPS:

- Australia
- Brazil
- Chile
- China
- Croatia
- Czech Republic
- Estonia

- Indonesia
- Japan
- Latvia
- Norway
- Russia
- Saudi Arabia
- South Korea
- Switzerland
- Taiwan
- Thailand
- Vietnam

In addition, a number of other counties and cities have taken stronger stances on GE foods. They include the following:

Australia—Ban or Moratorium on GMOs—New South Wales, South Australia, Tasmania, Victoria, Western Australia.

China—Ban or Moratorium on GMOs—Heilongjiang Province, Jilin Province, Liaoning Province.

India—Ban or Moratorium on GMOs—Punjab (and other northern states).

Italy—Ban or Moratorium on GMOs—Lazio Region, Marche Region, Molise Region, Tuscany Region. Italian cities: Brescia, Genoa, Milan, Rome, Turin.

Mexico—Proposed Ban on GMOs—Queretaro Province.

New Zealand—Ban or Moratorium on GMOs—Marlborough District, Napier, Waitakere City.

Philippines—Ban or Moratorium on GMOs—Bohol Province, Lloilo Province, South Cotabato Province, Valencia.

Spain—Ban or Moratorium on GMOs—Andalucia Region, Basque Region.

Switzerland—Ban or Moratorium on GMOs—Tessin Canton Province.

The United Kingdom—Ban or Moratorium on GMOs—

Cornwall County, Leicestershire County, North Radstock, South Gloucestershire, South Hams District, Wales, Warwickshire.

BEYOND NATIONAL BORDERS—ESTABLISHING INTERNATIONAL RULES FOR GENETICALLY ENGINEERED FOOD

In the age of globalization, international trade rules regarding new technologies have become more and more critical. Because countries are regulating genetically engineered foods differently, the establishment of common trade rules has been very difficult. In fact, establishing trade rules for genetically engineered foods is one of the most contentious international issues and often pits the U.S. government against much of the rest of the world. Genetically engineered foods were a major source of protests at the now infamous World Trade Organization (WTO) meeting in Seattle in early December 1999, as well as the most recent WTO meeting in Cancun, Mexico, in 2003.

The process of establishing international rules for genetically engineered foods is taking two tracks: one is through the WTO, and the other is through the United Nations Biosafety Protocol.

The WTO sets the rules for trade for its 146 nation participants. At the WTO meeting in Seattle, U.S. trade negotiators tried to open foreign markets for U.S. grown genetically engineered crops. The U.S. trade team viewed many of the anti-GE policies of foreign governments as unfair barriers to trade. However, other countries (including the European Union, Japan, and India) disagreed, and a compromise could not be worked out. In 2003, the Bush Administration raised the stakes for GE foods at the WTO meeting in Cancun. It filed a formal complaint with the WTO dispute resolution body to challenge the EU's moratorium on GE foods. That dispute will likely be decided sometime in 2004, and will have broad repercussions for the other 144 member nations of the WTO. Separately, the U.S. is expected to challenge the EU's labeling requirements for GE foods at the WTO level.

In September 2003, the UN's Biosafety Protocol went into full effect for the over 50 countries that have ratified a treaty, which says environmental, human health, and socioeconomic factors are recognized as valid considerations in determining whether to accept or reject GMO imports. The Protocol for the first time establishes on an international level that genetically engineered foods are distinct and different, and should be regulated differently than conventional foods. It will likely have a major impact on U.S. exports to nations participating in the treaty because although the U.S. is not a participant, participating nations can still enforce the treaty when handling imports from non-participating countries. Under the treaty, shipments containing genetically engineered commodities must be labeled that they "may contain" genetically modified organisms. Because there is not a good system for segregating GE from non-GE crops in the U.S., many U.S. corn, soybean, and cotton exports will likely require labels stating that they "may contain" GMOs. This may cause some nations to look to other countries besides the U.S. for these commodities.

It is unclear how the Biosafety Protocol will interact with the WTO on GE foods and crops. If the WTO rules in favor of the U.S. in its challenge of the EU's GE food policy, it is uncertain how the Biosafety Protocol would fit with that decision.

HOW DOES THE U.S. REGULATE GENETICALLY ENGINEERED FOODS?

IN 1992, the Food and Drug Administration issued a "Statement of Policy" that would forever change your food supply. The FDA initiative determined that genetically engineered foods were "substantially similar" to conventional crops, and thus were not required to be labeled or undergo special safety testing before they entered the marketplace.

The 1992 FDA policy opened the floodgates for over fifty different genetically engineered organisms to become part of the foods we eat every day—including over two thirds of soybeans, a third of the corn crop, and over 70 percent of all cotton, according to USDA. Other commercialized genetically engineered crops include canola, potatoes, squash, tomatoes, papaya, and sweet peppers, although tomatoes and potatoes have been subsequently pulled from the market. On the horizon is genetically engineered wheat.

Three agencies currently regulate genetically engineered products—the FDA (regulating food and drugs), U.S. Environmental Protection Agency (regulating pesticides), and U.S. Department of Agriculture (regulating farm production). Critics of the U.S. system argue that it utilizes outdated regulatory statutes designed to regulate non-GE foods and crops. The U.S. Congress has yet to pass a regulatory statute that deals specifically with the unique threats posed by genetically engineered crops and foods.

ARE GENETICALLY ENGINEERED FOODS TESTED FOR HUMAN HEALTH RISKS?

AS WE'VE mentioned previously, genetically engineered foods in the U.S. are not required to undergo specific safety tests prior to entering the market. While food additives are subjected to a rigorous round of testing, meeting the standard of "a reasonable certainty of no harm," the FDA has determined that the genetically engineered foods currently on the market do not qualify as additives.

Under the Food Drug and Cosmetic Act (FDCA) of 1958, if foods are "Generally Regarded As Safe" (GRAS) they are exempt from premarket review. The FDA has determined that genetically engineered foods introduced thus far fit the GRAS category.

From 1992–2000, when a biotech firm submitted a new product for approval, the company was "encouraged" to participate in the FDA's "voluntary" consultation process. As the FDA points out, every company that has placed a genetically engineered food product on the market has participated in the consultation process. But each company voluntarily submits different types of tests—and only the summary of the data, not the entire studiies are sent to the FDA. The tests are neither peer reviewed nor made available for public scrutiny. And the testing is largely done by the company seeking guidance from the agency. In January 2001, the FDA announced revised rules for regulating genetically engineered foods that essentially made the previous "voluntary" process mandatory. But the rules offer little new requirements from the old system—they still do not require mandatory compositional analysis, animal feeding tests, and long-term volunteer human feeding studies. In other words, mandatory consultations are required, but not mandatory testing.[1] And a 2003 report by the Center for Science in the Public Interest found that even on occasions where the FDA asked biotech companies to submit more testing data, companies like Monsanto, CIBA–Geigy (now Syngenta), and Dow AgroSciences declined to submit the requested scientific data.

As detailed in chapter 2, a particular health concern is the potential exposure to food allergens. Although the FDA cosponsored a scientific meeting on food allergies in genetically engineered foods in 1994, the agency has yet to develop and publish guidance to industry on how to assess the allergenic potential of new proteins.

"We know that there is some possibility that a new protein in food may be an allergen for some individuals," admits FDA biochemical engineer Tong-Jen Fu, Ph.D., who is working on methods to determine the allergenic potential of new proteins that may be introduced in food.[2]

"Most proteins added to foods via genetic engineering cannot be tested for allergenicity. Instead, industry scientists simply screen the biochemical characteristics of proteins to see if they are consistent with the characteristics associated with allergens. It remains to be seen how effective such screening will be in protecting public health," Dr. Rebecca Goldburg of Environmental Defense told an FDA panel.[3]

Another concern is the lack of toxicity testing. Dr. Puztai's important rat study with a strain of genetically engineered potato (see chapter 2) is one of the few rat animal feeding studies conducted on genetically engineered foods. "Currently, there is no requirement of toxicity testing to ensure genetically engineered substances are safe—what is needed is long-term rat studies," according to Jean Halloran of the Consumers Union.[4]

There is also no FDA screen for imported genetically engineered foods. Genetically engineered foods from other countries with even less regulations in place than the U.S., such as Argentina, Mexico, and China, may not have undergone any safety review before entering the U.S. "We have no clue about imported food," says Halloran. "There are active programs in many other countries—and will be more soon. They are growing everything there."[5]

CONTROVERSY WITHIN THE FDA
OVER ITS 1992 POLICY

WHEN THE FDA announced its 1992 policy, the agency argued that it was supported by a clear scientific consensus that genetically engineered crops were "substantially equivalent" to other crops. But as documents made public as a result of a recent lawsuit indicate, many of the FDA's own scientists strongly disagreed with the policy.

In a memo to FDA Biotechnology Coordinator James Maryanski in 1992, FDA compliance officer Dr. Linda Kahl argued that genetically engineered crops and traditional crops were not the same. "The process of genetic engineering and traditional breeding are different, and according to the technical experts in the agency, they lead to different risks," Dr. Kahl wrote.[6]

In a separate memorandum, Dr. Louis Pribyl, a FDA microbiologist, commented that a draft of the FDA policy "read very pro-industry, especially in the area of unintended effects." It is "industry's pet idea that there are no unintended effects that will raise the FDA's level of concern." But time and again, Prybil wrote, "there is no data to back up their contention."[7]

IS THE ENVIRONMENT BEING PROTECTED?

THE U.S. Environmental Protection Agency is in charge of protecting the environment from potential adverse effects of genetically engineered crops. But the agency has been sharply criticized by environmental groups and leading scientists for ignoring important environmental statutes, and allowing genetically engineered crops into the fields with little information on possible adverse environmental effects.

In a rare move, even an EPA scientific advisory panel told the agency in February 2000 that it needs to strengthen its oversight of new genetically engineered crops to ensure that they aren't harmful to insects and butterflies, including the Monarch butterfly. The advisory panel, an independent, peer review body, told the EPA that the crops should be tested on a wider variety of insects to determine their effects and that the EPA should require more data from seed companies on the impact of crops in the field.[8]

In 2002, a National Academy of Sciences report took the EPA to task for relying on too little data, and called some of its environmental assessments superficial. The NAS was critical of the EPA's cult of secrecy, shutting out the public from reviewing the agency's decisions. And the NAS report highlighted that the EPA was short on institutional knowledge in the area of environmental impacts, and does not do postmarket monitoring of genetically engineered crops. For example, the Cornell University study on the Monarch butterfly, and the New York University study on the engineered Bt remaining toxic in the soil (see chapter 3)—both clearly important studies with serious implications—were not required to be done at all by the EPA, let alone before the crops they studied enter the marketplace.

As we discussed in chapter 3, the EPA is currently being sued by Greenpeace, the Center for Food Safety, and numerous other environmental groups and organic farmers because of the way it has regulated crops with the genetically engineered Bt spliced into it. Among several charges, the lawsuit claimed that the EPA has ignored the Federal Fungicide, Insecticide and Rodenticide Act (FIFRA) and the National Environmental Policy Act (NEPA) by allowing Bt plants on the market.[9]

The lawsuit charged that the EPA has allowed genetically engineered Bt plants to enter the market despite recent research indicating that these engineered plants will speed up the development of pest resistance to natural Bt sprays (an important tool for organic farmers), transfer engineered Bt traits to like-weeds creating so-called "Superweeds," and have adverse impacts on beneficial insects and other non-target organizations. In addition, the EPA ignored a requirement under NEPA to prepare an environmental impact statement that analyzes the environmental, socioeconomic, and cumulative impacts of its program registering genetically engineered Bt plants. Unfortunately, federal courts refused to take Bt corn off the market, and the EPA gave approval for 7 more years of Bt crop cultivation in 2001.

A major battle is now brewing at the U.S. Department of Agriculture (USDA) regarding the introduction of GE wheat. A large coalition of family farm and environmental groups are demanding an Environmental Impact Statement (EIS), required under NEPA, be done before Monsanto's Roundup Ready wheat is introduced into the market. The groups have filed a legal petition with the USDA calling for the EIS to also include potential economic damages—as most major wheat buyers have said they will not import GE wheat if it is introduced into the U.S. The U.S. has lost considerable exports because Europe will not accept GE corn. Iowa State University economist Robert Wisner has estimated that prices for wheat could fall 35–50 percent if GE wheat is introduced, because of lost export markets.

ALTHOUGH GENETICALLY engineered Bt crops have been planted commercially in U.S. fields since 1995, it took the agency five years to put together guidelines for farmers to address the potentially catastrophic effects of pest resistance. Both the biotech industry and the EPA recognize that genetically engineered Bt crops will speed up the development of resistance to Bt by the major target pests—the pink bollworm (cotton) and the corn borer (corn)—in as few as three years (as we further detail in chapter 3). Pest resistance could mean a new strain of "superbugs" able to withstand pesticides.

Under current EPA rules, most farmers planting GE Bt corn are required to plant 20–25 percent of their crop as non-Bt corn—creating a kind of refuge. Farmers planting genetically engineered Bt cotton are required to plant 4–20 percent of non-engineered cotton. The EPA hopes that this will slow down the development of resistance to the Bt toxin by various pests—particularly the corn borer and pink bollworm.

Unfortunately the refuge plans are "based in large part on computer models and not on large-scale field experiments....Elements of the plans are highly controversial among entomologists and others who believe they are inadequate to forestall the evolution of resistant pests," says Rebecca Goldburg of Environmental Defense.[10] Even more troubling is the evidence that many farmers are not complying with the refuge requirements. A 2003 USDA survey found that approximately 20 percent of farms in 10 major agriculture states were not complying with the refuge requirements.[11]

Additionally, the new EPA rules have very weak enforcement provisions—requiring biotech seed companies to instruct farmers about the new rules and make sure they are complying. Biotech seed firms, not the EPA, are supposed to work with the farmers to report any adverse effects to Monarchs or other wildlife as a result of the genetically engineered crops.

WHO'S RESPONSIBLE FOR GENETIC CONTAMINATION?

THE THREAT of unknown genetically engineered pollen flying through the air to pollute another farmer's land is considered "one of the GM hot potatoes," according to Dr. Charles Benbrook[12] (see chapter 3 for more details). Already a major organic food company, Terra Prima, lost hundreds of thousands of dollars when it discovered that the organic corn it was using was contaminated.[13] But so far, neither the EPA or USDA are regulating problems associated with genetic drift, and there are no existing regulations to deal with it.

USDA'S TEST PLOTS

THE USDA'S primary responsibility in overseeing genetically engineered crops is through the approval of field trials. In this area, the USDA has acted essentially as a rubber stamp. According to a study by the U.S. Public Interest Research Group (USPIRG), from 1987 through 2002, the USDA authorized 15,461 field releases of genetically engineered organisms on 39,660 field test sites spanning 482,226 acres. The USDA has rejected only 3.5 percent of requests for such releases, denying requests for reasons such as incomplete applications or other minor paperwork errors. The USDA largely operates under a notification process in which developers simply let the USDA know they are conducting a field trial with tests. There is very little oversight or monitoring done. Even more disconcerting is that it is the USDA's responsibility to oversee the new generation of biopharm crops, as discussed in the next section.

The USDA is hardly an impartial observer when it comes to GE crops. The agency has spent tens of millions of dollars in researching and promoting biotech crops. The agency helped to develop the "Terminator" technology, which rendered GE seeds sterile, thereby protecting the technology for the biotech industry. The USDA's agricultural secretary Ann Veneman, has been a long-time supporter of biotechnology, serving on the board of the biotech company Calgene prior to the USDA. She has also aggresively pushed GE foods at the international level.

BIOPHARM AND TEST CROPS

THE USDA regulates biopharm crops under the Plant Protection Act. The USDA has authorized corporations such as Monsanto, DuPont, Dow, and Prodigene to conduct over 300 field tests of biopharm crops genetically engineered to produce pharmaceuticals, industrial chemicals, and other medical and industrial products, including a blood clotting agent, blood thinner, various blood proteins, experimental animal vaccines, industrial enzymes, antibodies, and an important abortion-inducing compound once considered for use as an AIDS drug.[14] None of these biopharm crops have been approved for human or animal consumption. Yet the USDA continues to allow these open-air tests to take place, in secret locations, without revealing the exact details of what is being grown. Of particular concern is that biopharm crops are typically corn or soybeans—GE crops that have frequently contaminated non-GE food crops.

The USDA's oversight of biopharm crops has come under heavy criticism from environmental groups and the scientific community. In 2002, the National Academy of Sciences issued a report calling for greater oversight, warning that the environmental impacts of biopharm crops cannot be predicted, and that the novel compounds may contaminate human and animal food supplies.

There have already been a few red flags related to biopharmed crops. In 2003, the EPA fined Dow AgroSciences and Pioneer

Hi-Bred International for failing to comply with permits to plant biopharm crops in Hawaii. In November 2002, the USDA announced that there had been biocontamination of food crops in Iowa and Nebraska involving test plots by the biotech company Prodigene.

In 2003, after years of pressure from environmental and consumer organizations, the U.S. Department of Agriculture announced improved oversight of field trials of new genetically engineered biopharmed crops and said that it would expand its staff from 33 to 50, not including federal inspectors already stationed in states. Among the new measures: greater distances separating pharm crops from regular crops, training for farmers, equipment dedicated to pharm crops, and more frequent government inspections. Under new cultivation rules, fields of pharmaceutical and industrial crops will be inspected seven times over a two-year period to ensure there is no contamination of conventional crops. And in January 2004, the USDA finally agreed to conduct an environmental impact assessment of biopharming, though it has no mandate to examine potential impacts on wildlife.

But environmental groups don't believe the USDA is going far enough. Because the contamination from GE crops to non-GE crops is so widespread, and currently difficult to control, it is likely that further contamination involving biopharm crops will take place. Environmental groups are calling for a ban on open-air cultivation of biopharm crops, the halt of using food crops in biopharming, and restricting testing to indoors.

The FDA does not regulate biopharm field trials, so the agency has been limited in its oversight of biopharm crops. Thus far, they have issued only recommendations, not regulations. For instance, the FDA has *not* prohibited use of pesticides on drug crops, has no clear protocols for allergenicity testing of these drugs, and leaves open a loophole for potential dual-use of biopharm crop residues for food or animal feed, according to Friends of the Earth.[15]

Interestingly enough, biopharm crops have exposed a division within the food industry and the biotech industry. For the first time, previous biotech supporters, the Grocery Manufacturers of America, and the National Food Processors Association, called for tougher regulations with regards to biopharmed crops in the wake of the Prodigene revelations. They are demanding a system of zero contamination—something that the biotech industry and USDA have not been able to guarantee.

REGULATING GE FISH

IN JANUARY 2004, Yorktown Technologies began selling the first genetically engineered fish in the U.S. The so-called "GloFish" is a pet fish that has been created by adding genes from a coral species to the genome of the common black-and-white zebra danio. Remarkably, the Food and Drug Administration has no policies to regulate pet GE fish.

There is concern that the introduction of the GloFish is the first step toward genetically engineered fish meant for human consumption. In 2002, more than 200 grocers, restaurants, and seafood distributors, representing 40 states (including the District of Columbia), publicly announced that they pledge not to purchase or sell genetically engineered fish. They were responding to an application filed with the FDA for market approval for genetically engineered salmon developed by Aqua Bounty Farms. Consumer and environmental groups have called for a ban on the introduction of GE fish until the ecological and human health risks are better understood. The National Academy of Sciences raised human health and environmental risks associated with GE fish, and particular GE salmon, in its 2002 report, "Animal Biotechnology: Identifying Science-based Concerns."

Currently, the FDA is in charge of approving GE fish, despite the obvious environmental implications of introducing a new species into aquatic environments. Because there are no GE-animal/fish specific regulations or laws, the FDA is regulating GE fish under federal drug laws.[16]

WHY IS THERE NO LABELING OF GENETICALLY ENGINEERED FOODS?

IF THE U.S. had comprehensive labeling of genetically engineered foods, this book would not have to be written. Despite nearly fifty different genetically engineered foods on the market, and approximately 90 percent of the public supporting labeling, the FDA has stuck by its 1992 decision not to label these radically new foods.

The FDA does not seem to hesitate to require or allow numerous other types of labels for food. For example, labeling for kosher products, sugar, artificial flavoring, salt, cholesterol, and preservatives are all required, and labels on orange and other juices must indicate whether they are from concentrate.

Yet, there is no labeling requirement for genetically engineered foods in the U.S. Under the Food, Drug, and Cosmetic Act, labeling is required when something is a "material fact" to consumers. The FDA has determined that in the case of genetically engineered foods, a "material fact" applies only when a food contains a known allergen, or decreases the nutritional value of the food.[17]

In objection to the FDA's labeling policy, the Center for Food Safety and the Alliance for Bio-Integrity filed a major lawsuit that brought together consumers, environmentalists, organic farmers, chefs, and religious leaders—all demanding that the FDA require labeling and safety testing of genetically engineered foods.

Members of the U.S. Congress have at times responded to the growing call for labeling. In November 1999, a letter signed by a bipartisan group of forty-seven members of Congress calling for the labeling of genetically engineered foods was sent to the Food and Drug Administration. The signers of the letter, circulated by House Minority Whip David Bonior (D-MI), disagreed with the FDA's interpretation of the Federal Food, Drug, and Cosmetic Act, arguing that the Act was intended to ensure that consumers are provided thorough information and are not misled about the characteristics of their food. The members of Congress who signed the letter asserted that the FDA is required to label genetically engineered or modified foods under current law.

In the meantime, Congressman Dennis Kucinich (D-OH) introduced the Genetically Engineered Food Right to Know Act, which would require mandatory labeling of genetically engineered foods. Senator Barbara Boxer (D-CA) introduced companion legislation on the Senate. The bills would also apply to animals fed genetically engineered material but would not require restaurants to comply with labeling. The label would read: "United States government notice: This product contains genetically engineered material, or was produced with a genetically engineered material."

The biotech and food industry have strongly opposed the Kucinich bill and all forms of mandatory labeling. The National Food Processors Association (NFPA) and the Alliance for Better Foods (funded by food trade associations) pushed for so-called voluntary industry labeling. And they won. In early 2002, as part of the FDA's revised rules, the agency set up guidelines for voluntary labeling of genetically engineered, or non-genetically engineered foods. Of course, voluntary labeling products as "GE-free" places extra costs and burdens on companies that choose not to use the technology. As predicted, voluntary GE-free labeling has been used only sporadically within the food industry. And no food companies have decided to label their products as "genetically engineered."

In 2003, Representative Kucinich went a step further and introduced a new comprehensive regulatory framework for genetically engineered foods and crops, which required labeling, pre-market testing, further research, and liability for biotech companies; allowed farmers to save seeds; and mandated stronger regulations for biopharm crops. Despite the strong bills introduced by Representative Kucinich, Congress has yet to enact a new regulatory bill for genetically engineered foods and animals.

WHILE REGULATORY activity has been slow to move forward at the federal level, a number of bills, initiatives, and resolutions have been introduced at the state and local levels. These efforts have struggled to find success, but they continue to pop up each year. Following are a few of the bills, initiatives, and resolutions that have been introduced:

State Bills
- In **California,** state legislators have introduced labeling legislation in the state senate.
- In **Nebraska,** a state senator has introduced a bill that would hold makers of genetically modified seeds liable for damages if the plants cross-pollinate with a neighbor's crops.
- In **Vermont,** state legislators have introduced a bill that would place a one-year moratorium on growing genetically engineered crops, while the effects of GE crops are studied further.
- In **Minnesota,** state legislators have introduced three separate bills: One would place a five-year moratorium on the planting of genetically engineered crops. The second would place liability of any environmental damage caused by engineered crops squarely on the seed companies—not farmers. And the final bill is a strict mandatory labeling bill.
- In **Michigan,** a strict labeling bill has been introduced at the state legislature.
- In **West Virginia,** a bill was introduced that would require any food served in schools to be GE free.
- In **Maryland,** the state has passed a moratorium on the release of genetically engineered aquatic species into waters flowing into the Chesapeake Bay in April 2001.
- In **New York** state, legislation was introduced calling for a five-year moratorium on the planting of genetically engineered crops beginning in the year 2001.

Local Initiatives and Resolutions

- **Mendocino County** in California voted to ban the growing of GE crops in their county in early 2004.
- In **Berkeley,** the City Council passed a resolution calling for federal labeling of genetically engineered foods in December 1999.
- In **Boston,** the City Council called for a moratorium in March 2000 on genetically engineered foods and crops until further testing is done. The council called for federal labeling for those that have been approved.
- Elsewhere in **Massachusetts,** the towns of Ashfield, Chesterfield, Plainfield, and Windsor have passed resolutions calling for a ban or moratorium on GMOs, and/or labeling of GE foods.
- In **Vermont,** the towns of Cabot, Calais, Charlotte, Chester, Fletcher, Greensboro, Hardwick, Jamaica, Johnson, Marshfield, Newark, Peru, Ripton, Rochester, Shoreharm, Walden, and Westfield have voted for a ban or moratorium on GMOs.

WHAT SHOULD BE LABELED?

THERE IS little debate that whole food crops, such as genetically engineered corn or potatoes, would be simple to label. But what about processed foods that contain ingredients made from genetically engineered plants such as canola oil, corn flour, cottonseed oil, or lecithin? And what percentage of genetically engineered material would trigger the need for a label?

Under the Kucinich bill, processed foods that contain .1 percent of genetically engineered material would have to be labeled as such. That is the lowest percentage at which foods can be reliably tested at the present time for genetically engineered material. Genetic ID, based in Iowa, was the world's first laboratory to offer GMO testing in 1996 and now licenses its DNA testing technique to laboratories around the world. Monsanto's Roundup Ready soybeans can be detected with a simple $5.75 protein-based test being sold by Strategic Diagnostics Inc. (SDI) of Newark, Delaware, which produces results in three to five minutes—acting similar to a home pregnancy test. SDI offers tests that can identify four popular varieties of genetically engineered Bt corn. (There are currently thirteen varieties of engineered corn on the market.) Maine-based EnviroLogix already makes a quick test for some GE foods.

There are still technical difficulties involved in testing for some processed foods—including, for example, corn flakes. Highly processed sugars and oils are also difficult to test because they have few proteins from which to extract DNA. The processing of products like corn syrup has helped serve as a cover for some food companies. For example, Coca-Cola tells consumers that it "does not use ingredients that are genetically modified."[20] But upon further questioning, the company argues that any genetically engineered ingredients they may use are destroyed in the processing. Coca-Cola will not guarantee that the corn used in its corn syrup is genetically engineered free.

Nevertheless, the issue of what constitutes a genetically engineered product, and what should require labeling, will likely be a hotly debated topic in the coming years.

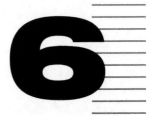

6

WHAT FOOD PRODUCTS, INGREDIENTS, AND COMPANIES SHOULD YOU AVOID?

HOW YOU CAN IDENTIFY GENETICALLY ENGINEERED FOOD

IF YOU want to avoid eating genetically engineered food, you will face several obstacles. The number-one hurdle is the lack of labeling. The absence of labeling muddles things at every step of the food chain. While a farmer knows whether his crops are genetically engineered, the companies that buy his harvest generally follow a "don't ask, don't tell" policy—although that is slowly changing. Until the point of purchase, genetically engineered crops and conventional crops are mixed together in giant grain elevators, as well as containers on trucks, train cars, barges, and ships—with possible contamination at each stage of the transportation chain.

Food companies that buy the crops as ingredients for their products then buy the mixed crop. And when there is once again no labeling on the final package, you along with the rest of American consumers are pretty much left in the dark.

To become an informed food detective, you are going to have to learn how to read labels, know what genetically engineered foods are on the market, and understand what ingredients are likely to have been made from genetically engineered crops. It will take diligence. But, as we discuss in chapters 7 and 8, finding food that is not genetically engineered is not only possible—it can have great rewards.

The most common genetically engineered foods are also staples in many of our diets: corn, soy, canola, dairy products, and cotton-seed oil, commonly used in vegetable oils. Thankfully, most of these genetically engineered foods are not in supermarkets in the form of whole foods, which are found in the produce section (although many of the foods in supermarket dairy cases come from cows injected with rBGH). In fact, most genetically engineered crops are used in animal feed or used as ingredients in processed foods—particularly corn, canola, and soy. It is estimated that at least 60 percent of processed foods on the market currently contain ingredients derived from genetically engineered soybeans alone.

In the ensuing pages, we will take you through some of the main genetically engineered foods and their derivative ingredients. Keep in mind that these ingredients will not be labeled as genetically engineered. However, because genetically engineered crops are intermingled with conventional crops, there is a good chance that they contain some genetically engineered material. The approach we outline in this book helps you identify foods that may be genetically engineered, and foods that you know are not. Armed with this information you should be able to dramatically decrease your consumption of genetically engineered foods and ingredients.

Canola (Rapeseed oil)

Chicory, red-hearted (Radicchio)

Corn—includes sweet corn and popcorn

Cotton

Flax

Papaya

Potato

Soybean

Squash

Sugarbeet

Tomato

Source: Union of Concerned Scientists[1]

GENETICALLY ENGINEERED FOODS AND DERIVATIVES

THE FIRST step is to simply commit to memory the crops listed, and know the numerous ingredients and derivatives that are commonly used in all kinds of processed foods that can find their way into your shopping cart.

Several large food companies, including Coca-Cola, have argued that ingredients made from genetically engineered crops should not constitute genetically engineered ingredients—or define their product as "genetically engineered." Coca-Cola claims that the DNA from any genetically engineered crops is destroyed during processing which creates oils, syrups, and other derivatives. However, there is evidence that this is not the case. According to Dr. Gordon Wiseman of RHM Technology in Buckinghamshire, UK, a company that tests for genetically engineered content in food, all soy lecithin and up to 50 percent of oil samples contain enough DNA to still test positive as being genetically engineered after processing.[2]

Below is a list of "prime suspects" of foods that have been genetically engineered. We have listed the whole food, derivatives, and common products that may contain these ingredients. Much of this information has been gathered by the nonprofit organization Mothers for Natural Law[3]:

- **Soybeans**—*Derivatives: lecithin, soybean oil, soy flour, soy protein, soy isolates, genistein.* Lecithin E322 is the most common additive in food. Used as an emulsifier, lecithin can be found in as much as 60 percent of all processed foods. Used in bread and bakery products, chocolate, margarine, cheese spread, mayonnaise, powdered milk and baby milk, cream, cheese spreads, fresh pasta, flan, mousses.[4] Products that may contain genetically engineered soy derivatives: vitamin E, tofu dogs, cereals, veggie burgers and sausages, tamari, soy sauce, chips, ice cream, frozen yogurt, infant formula, sauces, protein powder, margarine, soy cheeses, crackers, breads, cookies, chocolates, candies, fried foods, shampoo, bubble bath, cosmetics, enriched flours and pastas.
- **Corn**—*Derivatives: corn syrup, corn fructose, corn starch, corn dextrose, corn oil, corn flour.* Products that may contain genetically engineered corn derivatives: vitamin C, tofu dogs, chips, candies, ice cream, infant formula, salad dressings, tomato sauces, breads, cookies, cereals, baking powder, alcohol, vanilla, margarine, soy sauce, tamari, soda, fried foods, powdered sugar, enriched flours and pastas. There are several other food ingredients created from corn that are not easily identified as corn products. Those include the following:

    Dextrose, glucose, maltose, fructose, sucrose (syrups and solids)—Sugars processed from corn syrup used in sweet products like fruit and soft drinks.

    Maltodextrin—An industrial carbohydrate filler derived from corn. It's found in many processed foods such as gravy mixes and flavored chips, and used in cooked processed meats such as sliced ham and chicken, and in dry baby foods.[5]

Xanthan gum (E415)—Derived from corn sugar, a thickener in ice cream, salad dressings, and confectionery.

- **Canola**—*Derivatives: canola oil.* Products that may contain genetically engineered canola derivatives: chips, salad dressings, cookies, margarine, soaps, detergents, soy cheeses, fried foods.

- **Cotton**—*Derivatives: cottonseed oil, vegetable oil, cotton fabric.* Products that may contain genetically engineered cotton or its derivatives: clothes, linens, chips, peanut butter, crackers, cookies.

- **Potatoes**—*Derivatives: potato starch and flour.* The only genetically engineered potato variety is the Russet Burbank. Products that may contain genetically engineered potatoes or derivatives: unspecified processed or restaurant potato products (fries, mashed, baked, mixes, etc.), chips, Passover products, vegetable pies, soups.

- **Tomatoes**—No plum or roma tomatoes have been genetically engineered. But one variant of cherry tomato has, as have regular tomatoes. Products that may contain genetically engineered tomatoes or derivatives: sauces, purees, pizza, lasagna, and all processed Italian and Mexican foods.

- **Papaya**—Currently the only fruit genetically engineered. Others in development include: apples, grapes, strawberries, pineapples, bananas, melons.

- **Crook-necked yellow squash**—Can be found in whole form, or in some baby foods.

- **Dairy products**—Milk, cheese, butter, buttermilk, sour cream, yogurt, whey. Milk from cows injected with the recombinant Bovine Growth Hormone (rBGH) is mixed together with conventionally produced milk, creating an identification problem similar to other genetically engineered crops. Find out more about GE-free dairy products in chapter 7. Cheese poses some unique problems. Several types of rennet are used for making cheese—including GE versions called chymosin or chymax, as well as animal rennet. The term "microbial enzyme" on a cheese package may refer to vegetable rennet (a natural enzyme from a mold), but this term is also used for genetically engineered rennet. "Vegetarian cheeses" may also contain genetically engineered rennet or vegetable rennet. According to the Consumers Union, some 60 percent of all hard cheese products in the U.S. are made with an engineered form of rennet.

SPECIFIC GENETICALLY ENGINEERED INGREDIENTS

ASIDE FROM genetically engineered whole foods, there are a number of specific ingredients that have been genetically engineered. The list below names the ingredient and some common products where it is used.[6]

- **Aspartame** (also known as NutraSweet)—a genetically engineered chemical that is usually found in diet soft drinks—but is also in over 9,000 products, including children's vitamins and medicines; chewing gum; many low-fat products, such as jelly, jam, and yogurt; and some candy.
- **Baker's yeast**—Genetically engineered yeast has been on the market for several years. It has been engineered to speed up the production of enzymes responsible for dough fermentation.
- **Brewer's yeast**—Used primarily in beer, it has an enzyme that makes it produce more alcohol. It is unclear how frequently it is used.
- **Riboflavin** (Vitamin B2)—Engineered to increase the bacteria production of riboflavin; has an antibiotic resistance marker. It is used to fortify or enhance nutritionally many processed foods such as baby foods, breakfast cereals, fruit drinks, and vitamin-enriched milk, and is also found in vitamin supplements.

- **Alpha amylase**—An enzyme that breaks down starch-producing more sugars for the starch to work—used in cereals, soft drinks, beer, and wine.
- **Hemicellulase**—Used to improve the strength of gluten in bread flour.
- **Lipase and triaclyglycerol**—Genetically engineered enzyme used to break down fats—could be used in the manufacture of margarine, chocolate, and baked goods.

FOODS TESTING POSITIVE

THERE HAS been no comprehensive testing of all food products on the market to find out which have genetically engineered ingredients—and which don't. However, there have been several random samplings of commonly found food products. The major sampling was done in September 1999 by the highly respected Consumers Union, publisher of *Consumer Reports*.[7] The *New York Times*, Greenpeace, and Friends of the Earth have also paid for similar testing.

Listed here are food products that have tested positive for genetically engineered ingredients based on sampling by the above three sources. Keep in mind that the food industry estimates that 60–75 percent of all processed food in U.S. supermarkets likely contains genetically engineered ingredients:

- Alpo Dry Pet Food
- Aunt Jemima Pancake Mix
- Ball Park Franks
- Betty Crocker Bac-Os Bacon Flavor Bits
- Boca Burger Chef Max's Favorite
- Bravos Tortilla Chips
- Duncan Hines Cake Mix
- Enfamil ProSobee Soy Formula
- Frito-Lay Fritos Corn Chips

- Gardenburger
- General Mills Total Corn Flakes Cereal
- Green Giant Harvest Burgers
- Heinz 2 Baby Cereal
- Jiffy Corn Muffin Mix
- Kellogg's Corn Flakes
- Kraft's Balance Bars
- Light Life Gimme Lean
- McDonald's McVeggie Burgers
- Morning Star Farms Better 'n Burgers
- Nabisco Snackwell's Granola Bars
- Nabisco Snackwell's Snack Crackers
- Nestle Carnation Alsoy Infant Formula
- Old El Paso Taco Shells
- Ovaltine Malt Powdered Beverage Mix
- Post Blueberry Morning Cereal
- Quaker Chewy Granola Bars
- Quaker White Cheddar Corn Cakes
- Quaker Yellow Corn Meal
- Quick Loaf Bread Mix
- Shake 'n Bake mix, the crispy chicken nuggets variety
- Similac Isomil Soy Formula
- Taco Bell Taco Shells
- Tombstone Pizza
- Ultra Slim Fast

FOOD COMPANIES TESTING POSITIVE FOR GENETICALLY ENGINEERED INGREDIENTS

MOST MAJOR U.S. food companies are using genetically engineered foods, ingredients or derivatives. If they haven't taken specific steps to source GE-free crops, then they are buying crops that have been genetically engineered.

As you will read in chapter 7, a growing number of companies are going GE-free. This means that their entire brand-name product line is free of genetically engineered ingredients. Below is a list of food companies whose products have tested positive for genetically engineered ingredients. Food companies buy ingredients in bulk. If one product is found to contain genetically engineered ingredients, it is likely that those same ingredients are being used in the company's other products.

- Crisco
- Frito, Dorito, Tostito
- Green Giant
- Isomil and ProSobee
- Kellogg's
- Kraft
- McDonald's
- Nabisco
- Nestle
- Old El Paso
- Ovaltine
- Parkay
- Pillsbury
- Procter & Gamble
- Quaker Mills
- Wesson

Source: Consumer Reports, September 1999, *NYT,* 9-8-99.

GE-FREE IN OTHER COUNTRIES, BUT NOT IN THE UNITED STATES

Thus far, no major U.S. food companies have decided to not use genetically engineered ingredients in all their products, although some have taken small steps forward. This is frustrating for many U.S. consumers because many of these same companies have pledged to go GE-free in Europe.

Here are a list of some of the food companies that have gone GE-free in some countries or all of Europe, but have not done so in the U.S.:

- Coca-Cola
- General Mills
- Heinz
- Hershey's
- Kellogg's
- Kraft
- McDonald's
- Burger King
- Nabisco
- Nestle
- PepsiCo
- Pillsbury
- Procter & Gamble
- Quaker Oats
- Safeway
- Tengelmann (majority owner of A&P Supermarkets)

THE TWENTY-FIVE LARGEST
U.S. FOOD COMPANIES

NEARLY ALL of the largest food companies in the U.S. have refused to take steps to confirm that they are not using genetically engineered foods. In fact, the top 100 U.S. food companies all appear to be using genetically engineered ingredients in their foods. The environmental organization Friends of the Earth has contacted all of the top 100 companies and asked whether they are using genetically engineered ingredients. Most of the 100 have refused to comment.

Here is a list of the top twenty-five U.S. food companies based on Fortune magazine rankings, their contact information, and primary food products.[8] While not all of the companies responded to our requests for their position on genetically engineered foods, many did. Coca-Cola argued that any genetically engineered ingredients they may be using are destroyed in the processing. Frito-Lay pointed out that 95 percent of the corn they use is GE-free, but could not vouch for the rest of their ingredients. And Dole states that none of the fruit and vegetables they use are genetically engineered, however, it does not label its products GE-free, and doesn't confirm that other ingredients such as sweeteners are GE-free. We've listed abbreviated versions of company statements below. Please keep in mind that corporate leaders change jobs and policies all the time. We have made every effort to ensure that the information below is correct at the present time. We encourage you to contact the company directly for their latest position on GE foods.

1. Altria Group (owner of Kraft Foods)

Betsy Holden, President & CEO

3 Lakes Dr.

Northfield, IL 60093

Phone: 1–800–323–0768

Fax: 847–646–2922

Web sites: www.altria.com, www.kraftfoods.com

BRANDS: Kool-Aid, Maxwell House Coffee, Di Giorno, Stove Top, Oven Classics, Toblerone, Country Time Lemonade, Cheez-Whiz, Jell-O, Kraft Mayonnaise, Miracle Whip, Post Cereals, Nabisco Products.

COMPANY STATEMENT: "A significant percentage of corn and soy crops grown in the U.S. have been enhanced using biotechnology. So it's likely that some of our products do contain biotech ingredients from these crops. It's important to know there is broad scientific consensus that biotech foods and ingredients are safe."

2. ConAgra Inc.

Bruce Rohde, Chairman & CEO

One ConAgra Drive,

Omaha, NE 61802-5001

Phone: 402–595–4000 (General), 1–800–323–9985 (Healthy Choice Consumer Line)

Web site: www.conagrafoods.com

BRANDS: Montfort, La Choy, Swiss Miss, Healthy Choice, Hunts, Butterball, Orville Redenbacher's, Eckrich, Wesson.

3. PepsiCo Inc. (owner of Frito-Lay)

Roger A. Enrico, Chairman & CEO

700 Anderson Hill Road

Purchase, NY 10577

Phone: 914–253–2000

Fax: 914–253–2070

Web sites: www.pepsico.com, www.quakeroats.com

BRANDS: Pepsi, Frito-Lay, Quaker, Tropicana & PBG, Cheetos, Grandma's Cookies, Sun Chips, Aquafina, Alegro, Aunt Jemima, Cap'n Crunch, Life, Golden Grain, Gatorade, Noodle-Roni, Quaker Rice & Popcorn Cakes, Rice-A-Roni.

Frito-Lay (owned by PepsiCo)

Steven S. Reinemund, CEO

7701 Legacy Drive

Plano, TX 75024

Phone: 972–334–7000

Web site: www.fritolay.com

BRANDS: Cheetos Cheese Flavored Snacks, Cracker Jack, Doritos Tortilla Chips, Fritos Corn Chips, Funyuns, Onion Flavored Rings, Grandmas Cookies.

COMPANY STATEMENT: "Now that there is a renewed interest in biotechnology and some consumer confusion exists, we did not feel it appropriate to ask our growers to include Bt crops in what they sell us. At the same time, we have no plans to market or advertise any claim of 'Genetically Modified-Free' products. . . . Since we are also a large buyer of agricultural commodities, and more than a quarter of the North American crop is derived from biotechnology, just like other food companies, we could have biotechnology ingredients in our products."

4. Coca-Cola Enterprises Inc.

Douglas Ivestor, Chairman & CEO

P.O. Box 723040

Atlanta, GA 31139

Phone: 770–989–3000

Fax: 770–989–3640

Web site: www.cocacola.com

BRANDS: Coke, Fanta, Fruitopia, Minute Maid, Nestea, Powerade.

COMPANY STATEMENT: "The Coca-Cola Company does not use ingredients that are genetically modified." When asked for further clarification, a consumer affairs specialist said that any genetically engineered ingredients that the company might use are destroyed in the processing.

5. Archer Daniels Midland

G. Allen Andreas, Chairman & CEO

4666 Faries Parkway

Decatur, IL 62526

Phone: 800–637–5843

Web site: www.admworld.com

BRANDS: ADM is a leader in providing ingredients to other food companies. They produce baking aids and mixes, cocoa and chocolate, flours, oils and fats, and sweeteners.

6. Tyson Foods

John Tyson, Chairman & CEO

Tyson Foods, Inc.

P.O. Box 2020

Springdale, AR 72765–2020

Phone: 1–800–347–7675

Web site: www.tysonfoodsinc.com

BRANDS: Tyson Meats, American Favorite, Butcher Boy, Fred's IBP, Supreme Lean, Wilson's Food Service, Wilson's Continental Deli, Thorn Apple Valley.

COMPANY STATEMENT: "Tyson Foods does not currently distinguish between GMO and non-GMO when purchasing grain and meal for the purpose of blending animal feed with the exception of certified organic grain, which is used in the production of our Nature's Farm organic chicken line."

7. Sara Lee Corp.

John Bryan, Chairman & CEO
3 First National Plaza
Chicago, IL 60602
Phone: 312–274–8200, 1–800–323–7117 (customer service)
Fax: 312–274–8829
Web site: www.saralee.com
BRANDS: Ball Park, Hillshire Farm, Jimmy Dean, Sara Lee.

8. H. J. Heinz Company

William Johnson, President & CEO
600 Grant St.
Pittsburgh, PA 15219
Phone: 412–456–5700, 1–800–872–2229 (Heinz Baby Food Consumer Relations)
Fax: 412–456–6128
Web site: www.heinz.com
BRANDS: Budget Gourmet, Heinz, Ore-Ida, Starkist, Weight Watchers, Heinz baby food, Heinz Ketchup.
COMPANY STATEMENT: "Heinz has responded to concerns about GMOs throughout the world and will continue to be responsive to changes in consumer expectations as well as regulatory policy. We seek to avoid ingredients from GM sources. For example, in the case of tomatoes, we only use tomatoes bred utilizing traditional breeding technology. Additionally, we are working with non-tomato ingredient suppliers to understand the source of these ingredients and the future of the supply."

9. Dean Foods

Gregg L. Engles, Chairman & CEO
2515 McKinney Ave., Ste. 1200, Lock Box 30
Dallas, TX 75201
Phone: 214–303–3400, 800–431–9214
Fax: 214–303–3499
Web site: www.deanfoods.com

BRANDS: Dairy Brands, International Delight, Mocha Mix, Second Nature, Naturally Yours, Lactaid, Berkeley Farms, Carnation Coffee Mate Liquid, Dairy Ease, Hillside, Meadow Brook, VeriFine.

10. Kellogg Company

Carlos M. Gutierrez, CEO
One Kellogg Square, P.O. Box 3599
Battle Creek, MI 49016
Phone: 616–961–2000 (consumer affairs)
Fax: 616–961–2871
Web site: www.kelloggs.com

BRANDS: Apple Jacks, Cocoa Krispies, Corn Flakes, Crackel 'n Oat Bran, Special K, Raisin Bran, Just Right, Rice Krispies, PopTarts, Lender's Bagels, Eggo

COMPANY STATEMENT: "Kellogg Company uses grain from a number of suppliers in our country, so our supply would likely include biotechnology-produced grain in the same proportion that it occurs in the United States supply."

11. General Mills

Stephen Sanger, CEO
Number One General Mills Blvd.
Minneapolis, MN 55440
Phone: 612–540–2311, 1–800–328–1144 (consumer line)
Web site: www.generalmills.com

BRANDS: Pillsbury, Bisquick, Bugles, Fruit Roll-Ups, Gold Medal, Betty Crocker, Nature Valley, Yoplait, Colombo, Pop

Secret, Bac-Os, Golden Grahams, Cheerios, Cocoa Puffs, Chex, Fiber One, Total, Cinnamon Toast Crunch, Wheaties, Oatmeal Crisp, Pop-Secret, Raisin Nut Bran, Trix, Green Giant, Häagen-Däzs, Hungry Jack, Old El Paso, Progresso.

COMPANY STATEMENT: "Because of the growing use of biotechnology by farmers and the way that grain gets commingled in storage and shipment, it's certainly possible that some of our products may contain ingredients that have been improved through biotechnology."

12. Smithfield Foods Inc.

Joseph W. Luter III, Chairman & CEO
200 Commerce Street
Smithfield, VA 23430
Phone: 888–366–6767
Web site: www.smithfieldfoods.com
BRANDS: Gwaltney, Lykes, Smithfield Premium, Peyton's, Jamestown.

13. Campbell Soup Company

David Johnson, President & CEO
1 Campbell Place
Camden, NJ 08103
Phone: 856–342–4800 (1–800–257–8443)
Fax: 856–342–3878
Web site: www.campbellsoup.com
BRANDS: 75 percent of U.S. soup market, Franco-American, Godiva, Hungry-Man, Pace, Pepperidge Farm, Prego, SpaghettiOs, V8.

COMPANY STATEMENT: "The current U.S. supply of corn and soybeans includes a mix of genetically and non-genetically modified crops. Campbell's use of genetically modified ingredients is restricted primarily to this supply of corn and soybeans."

14. Land O' Lakes

Jack Gherty, CEO
P.O. Box 64101
St. Paul, MN 55164
Phone: 800–328–4155
Web sites: www.landolakes.com/
BRANDS: Land O'Lakes butter, cheese, sour cream, and milk.
COMPANY STATEMENT: "The majority of the food manufactured in the U.S. does not differentiate between GMO and non-GMO components. At this time, Land O'Lakes Inc. follows that practice."

15. Dole Food Co. Inc.

David Murdock, Chairman & CEO
P.O. Box 5132
Westlake Village, CA 91359–5132
Phone: 818–879–6600, 1–800–232–8888 (consumer center)
Fax: 818–879–4893
Web site: www.dole.com
BRANDS: Classic Salad, Complete Salad, Fruit Bowls, Lunch for One, Special Blends.
COMPANY STATEMENT: "Dole understands and respects the rights of consumers to choose whether the food they eat is derived from genetic engineering or from traditional plant breeding techniques. . . . Dole currently does not have any products that are genetically modified."

16. Hershey Foods Corp.

Kenneth Wolfe, Chairman & CEO
100 Crystal A. Drive
Hershey, PA 17033
Phone: 717–534–4200, 1–800–468–1714 (Consumer Relations)
Web site: www.hersheys.com
BRANDS: chocolate confectionary, non-chocolate confectionary, chips, drinks, ice-cream toppings, Almond Joy, 5th

Avenue, Cadbury's Candies, Caramellos, Chocolate Chips, Good + Plenty, Heath Bar, Hershey's Jolly Rancher, Kisses, KitKat, Milk Duds, Reese's, Oh Henry, Whoppers.

17. Hormel Foods Corp.

Joel Johnson, Chairman, President & CEO
One Hormel Place
Austin, MN 55912
Phone: 507–437–5611, 1–800–523–4635 (Consumer Affairs)
Fax: 507–437–5129 (Administration), 507–437–9852 (consumer affairs)
Web site: www.hormel.com
BRANDS: Fast 'N Easy, Homeland, Light Lean, Little Sizzlers, Old Smokehouse, Sandwich Maker, Wranglers, Dinty Moore, Chi-Chi's, Jennie-O, El Torito.
COMPANY STATEMENT: ". . . there have been a variety of developments in plant genetics that have significantly improved crop productivity and food quality . . . innovation and advancements in technology are a very important part of our mission and our responsibility to you as a valued customer. Hormel Foods will, therefore, continue to support the crop and vegetable industries' efforts to provide the safest and highest quality products available."

18. Interstate Bakeries Corp. (IBC)

James R. Elsesser, CEO
12 East Armour Blvd.
Kansas City, MO 64141
Phone: 816–502–4000
Web site: www.interstatebakeriescorp.com
BRANDS: Wonder, Hostess, Dolly Madison, Merita, Butternut, Drakes.

19. WM Wrigley Jr.

William Wrigley Jr., CEO

410 N. Michigan Avenue
Chicago, IL 60611
Phone: 312–644–2121
Web site: www.wrigley.com
BRANDS: Wrigley Spearmint, Doublemint, Juicy Fruit, Big Red, Alpine.

20. Pilgrim's Pride
O. B. Goolsby, Jr., CEO
P.O. Box 93
Pittsburg, TX 75686
Phone: 800–824–1159
Web site: www.pilgrimspride.com
BRANDS: Pilgrim's Pride Buffalo Wings, Chicken, and Eggs.

21. Chiquita Brands International
Fernando Aguirre, CEO
250 East Fifth Street
Cincinnati, OH 45202
Phone: 513–784–8000
Web site: www.chiquita.com
BRANDS: Chiquita bananas, pineapples, watermelon, strawberries, grapes.
COMPANY STATEMENT: "We do not sell any genetically modified bananas, nor do we market any other genetically modified fresh fruits or vegetables."

22. McCormick
Robert Lawless, CEO
18 Loveton Circle
Sparks, MD 21152–6000
Phone: 800–632–5847
Web site: www.mccormick.com
BRANDS: McCormick Chili Mixes, McCormick Spices, Grilling Sauces, Marinades, Gravy, Pastas, Old Bay.

COMPANY STATEMENT: "Based on the best information available, pure spices and herbs, such as black pepper and cinnamon, do not contain food ingredients developed through biotechnology. Due to the growing use of food ingredients developed through biotechnology and the way grain gets commingled in storage and shipment, some of our seasoning blends may contain ingredients that have been modified through biotechnology."

23. Corn Products International
Samuel C. Scott, CEO
5 Westbrook Corporate Center
Westchester, IL 60154
Phone: 708–551–2600
Web site: www.cornproducts.com
BRANDS: Sweeteners (glucose), starches, corn oil and gluten, dextrin, emulsifiers.
COMPANY STATEMENT: "Corn refiners rely on their ability to purchase large amounts of commodity grain from widespread sources throughout the corn-growing regions of the United States. Consequently, it is not possible to commercially guarantee that no corn from EU-unapproved varieties will enter the commercial grain system or be offered to corn wet-milling locations."

24. Gold Kist
Doug Reeves, Chairman of the Board
P. O. Box 2210
Atlanta, GA 30301
Phone: 1–866–GKFARMS
Web site: www.goldkist.com
BRANDS: Gold Kist Farms Chicken and Pork.

25. Flowers Industries
Amos R. McMullian, Chairman & CEO
1919 Flowers Circle

Thomasville, GA 31757
Phone: 912–226–9110
Web site: www.flowersfoods.com
BRANDS: Keebler, Cheez-It, Famous Amos, Hydrox, Mrs. Smith's, Nature's Own, Sunshine, Vienna Fingers.

BABY FOODS AND HOSPITAL FEEDING

THE ONLY analysis done in the U.S. on baby food and hospital/nursing home food was commissioned by Greenpeace in 1999.[9] The findings revealed the presence of transgenic DNA from genetically engineered foods in several popular brands of baby foods and in nutritional supplements used for tube feeding in hospitals and nursing homes.

Gerber Mixed Cereal for Baby, a dry three-grain cereal mix for infants, tested positive for DNA from transgenic insect-resistant "Bt" corn and herbicide-tolerant "Roundup Ready" (RR) soybeans. Shortly after the findings of the study were announced, Gerber announced that it would go GE-free and substitute organic ingredients in its baby food. Heinz also announced that its baby food would be GE-free. Additionally, while Enfamil, the baby formula company, has announced that it is going GE-free, Nestle and Ross Nutrition (maker of Similac) will continue to use genetically engineered ingredients.

The two nutritional supplements produced by Novartis' IsoSource and Ross Products' Osmolite both contained transgenic DNA from RR soy.

VITAMINS AND SUPPLEMENTS

GENETICALLY ENGINEERED ingredients have found their way into supplements. Many of the source materials used to produce the most common vitamins are food commodities such as soy and corn. The proteins of the soy or corn remain intact throughout the vitamin-making process. For instance, vitamin C is made with corn fructose—which may be genetically altered.

Because of these concerns, the National Nutritional Foods Association (NNFA), which represents retailers and manufacturers of dietary supplements, natural foods, and other products, recently filed a citizen petition with the FDA, demanding that the agency strengthen its evaluation process of genetically engineered foods and calling for more rigorous oversight of the new products. NNFA has also called for the labeling of GE foods. The NNFA wants to help manufacturers and consumers know more about genetically engineered ingredients in supplements.

RESTAURANTS

CONSUMERS ARE particularly vulnerable when it comes to genetically engineered foods in many restaurants. Restaurants are not required to label their food, and many chefs may not know whether their ingredients are genetically engineered or not. Most major fast food restaurants such as McDonald's and Burger King have told customers in Europe that they do not use genetically engineered ingredients. While no chain restaurants have made the same claim in the U.S., there is second-hand evidence that McDonald's, Burger King, and Wendy's have requested that their potatoes used for fries not be genetically engineered. (Find out more about efforts by chefs to go GE-free in chapter 7.) The Wall Street Journal reported in late April 2000 that McDonald's, Burger King, Frito-Lay, and Procter and Gamble have told their potato suppliers that they do not want genetically engineered potatoes.[10] Thus far, none of the fast food chains are labeling their potatoes as GE-free—perhaps hoping to not draw attention to other genetically engineered ingredients such as canola and soy. As listed earlier in this chapter, McDonald's veggie burger has already tested positive for containing genetically engineered ingredients—most likely soy. Also supporting the contention that the big three fast food chains are using GE-free potatoes was the statement by the Canadian company McCain's, the largest supplier of potatoes for french fries to fast food chains, that it would not use genetically engineered potatoes.[11]

7

WHICH COMPANIES AND STORES ARE GOING GE-FREE?

IN EUROPE, almost every major food manufacturer and supermarket chain has banned genetically engineered ingredients from its brand-name products (see chapter 5 for a country-by-country overview). This means that they will not sell genetically engineered foods, or ingredients derived from genetically engineered crops. Up until now, other than organic companies, very few U.S. food companies or supermarkets have banned the use of genetically engineered foods or ingredients for their brand-name products. Several supermarket chains, including Safeway, Shaw's, and Albertsons, have banned genetically engineered foods in their European stores, but have decided not to do so in the U.S.

But leaders of a new wave of popular natural and organic food stores have taken a stand. In December 1999, Whole Foods and Wild Oats, the two largest natural-food supermarket chains in the country, announced that they would ban the use of genetically engineered ingredients in their own brand-name food products and would pressure their suppliers to eliminate gene-altered ingredients from their product lines. Wild Oats labels their food as GE-free. This does not mean that all food products in these stores will not include genetically engineered ingredients—only that their store brands do not. Whole Foods has more than 600 products carrying its brand name. Wild Oats has about 700 products under its own brand.

"It's really not my position to say genetically engineered is a good thing or a bad thing," said Jim Lee, president and chief operating officer of Wild Oats. "It's a matter of having a shopping choice. A high percentage of our customers are opposed to anything artificially introduced into their food."[1]

In November 2002, another natural food supermarket chain, Trader Joe's, announced that it had successfully removed GE ingredients from most of its in-store products. Campaigns are being led through the True Food Network and Greenpeace targeting Safeway and Shaw's to get them to take similar steps toward removing GE products and ingredients from their stores.

Be on the look out for similar policies to be adopted at other major supermarket chains as consumer awareness about genetically engineered foods grows.

WHAT ABOUT FOOD COMPANIES?

WHILE MOST major traditional U.S. supermarkets have been slow to act, several food companies have made certain specific products GE-free.

- Both Heinz's Earth's Best line and Gerber—two of the biggest baby-food makers—announced in 1999 that they would try to make their products GE-free, and Gerber went a step further, declaring that it would substitute corn flour and soy flour that is "organic." The Gerber decision, in response to a letter from Greenpeace, was particularly important, given that the company is the largest baby-food manufacturer in the country as well as being a subsidiary of Novartis—the giant Swiss-based biotech company.[2]

- In March 2000, Mead Johnson Nutritionals, maker of Enfamil baby formula, announced that it would go GE-free. Enfamil is one of the nation's largest producers of baby formulas. Prior to this announcement it was impossible to get GE-free baby formula in the U.S.

- Kraft has been the target of a concerted consumer campaign by Friends of the Earth, U.S. PIRG, and others to stop using GE ingredients. Details on the campaign can be found at www.krafty.org. In 2002, the Genetically Engineered Food Alert coalition tested four Kraft products for the presence of genetically engineered corn, and found none of them contained it. This is especially significant since laboratory tests commissioned by the coalition ten months earlier found six products that contained genetically engineered corn. It appears that Kraft may be phasing out the use of genetically engineered corn in response to consumer concern and the risks highlighted by the StarLink corn contamination of Kraft products. Product samples that lab results indicated did not contain engineered corn were: Post Honey Bunches of Oats with Strawberries, Post Alpha Bits, Fig Newtons, and Barnum's Animal Crackers. Like several other big food companies, Kraft recently announced it will produce an organic line of food products that will be GE-free.

- In late April 1999, the Wall Street Journal uncovered what had been rumored for many months, that several major food companies were asking for non-GE potatoes. J.R. Simplot Co., a major supplier of french fries to McDonald's, is instructing its farmers to stop growing genetically engineered Bt potatoes. JR Simplot was told not to grow the GE spuds by several companies, including McDonald's, Burger King,

Frito-Lay, and Procter and Gamble. "Virtually all the [fast food] chains have told us they prefer to take nongenetically modified potatoes," Fred Zerza, spokesman for J. R. Simplot, told the Journal.[3]

- In October 1999, Hain Food Group Inc. announced that it would switch the oil it uses in its fryers from corn to safflower, and place labels on its Little Bear line of natural snacks, indicating that it contained no genetically engineered ingredients.[4]
- Worthington Foods Inc., which makes Morningstar Farms veggie burgers, announced in late 1999 that it would take genetically engineered soybeans out of its product.[5]
- Seagrams, one of the world's largest distillers, is telling farmers that it will not purchase genetically engineered corn.[6]
- Archer Daniels Midland, one of the world's largest suppliers of corn and soybean products, opened its first organic processing facility in 2003 for its NutriSoy® Organic Whole Soybean Powder.[7]

Other major natural and organic food companies that have made public statements indicating that they have gone GE-free include:

- Annie's Naturals
- Barbara's Bakery
- Eden's
- Lightlife Foods
- GeniSoy
- White Wave
- Northern Soy
- Walnut Acres
- Newman's Own
- SunRich
- Guiltless Gourmet
- Nature's Path

- Organic Valley
- Vitasoy
- Kettle Foods
- Pacific Grain and Foods

Source: Company Correspondence, People's Earth Network

The movement toward GE-free ingredients and products is very challenging for some food companies, particularly because of problems related to contamination. However, as major food companies jump on the organic bandwagon they are starting to stock and source more and more GE-free food products. A tremendous resource for food companies and suppliers looking for GE-free products is the newsletter Non-GMO Source (www.nongmosource.com). It also has a 2004 direct of sources, suppliers, and companies going GE-free.

For consumers, the True Food Network has an excellent, up-to-date shopper's guide on GE-free foods. It is available on the web at www.truefoodnetwork.org. The nonprofit Mothers for Natural Law also has an exhaustive list of products that are GE-free (www.safe-food.org).

COMPANIES BY TYPE OF PRODUCT

BELOW IS a list of companies that have stated that they do not use genetically engineered ingredients. This list, largely put together by Mothers for Natural Law, can be easily searched by food product.

- Flours—Arrowhead Mills; Eden flours.
- Sweeteners—Eden Organic Malted Grain Sweeteners, Kogee Organic Cane Sugar, Organic Cane Sugar, Pure USA Hone, Sucanat North America.
- Syrups—Eden Organic Malted Grain Sweeteners, Wholesome Foods Organic Backstrap Molasses, Andersons

Pure Maple Syrup, Cary's Maple Syrup (premium), Hauke Honey Pure Maple Syrup, Spring Tree Pure Maple Syrup.

- Olive oils (extra virgin)—Alessi Olio, Da Vinci, Eden Selected, Filippo Berio, Gourmet Aritrian, Grey Poupon, L'estronell, Odd Monk, Olitalia, Peloponnese, Spectrum Natural, Tassos.

- Other oils—Eden (organic sesame, toasted sesame, hot pepper toasted sesame, and safflower oils), Sigg Grapeseed Oil, Olitalia Grapeseed Oil, Loriva Sesame Oil, Spectrum Natural (almond oil, apricot kernel oil, avocado oil, coconut oil, safflower oil, walnut oil).

- Vinegars—Da Vinci Balsamic, Eden Apple Cider, L'estronell River Run Hot Pepper, Spectrum Organic (raspberry wine, red wine, white wine).

- Salad dressings and condiments—Cross and Blackwell Capers, Spectrum Zesty Italian Dressing, Jaffa Gold Lemon Juice, Melinda Extra Hot Sauce, Annie's Farmhouse Maple Mustard, Earth Fire Products Chutney, Eden Organic Mustard (and imported condiments), Sandhill Mustard, Santa Barbara Olive Company California Ripe Large or Jumbo Pitted Olives, Muir Glen Organic Tomato Ketchup, Cascadian Farm Organic Sauerkraut, Eden Organic Sauerkraut, Krinos Imported Grape Leaves.

- Nut and fruit butters—Arrowhead Mills (certified organic peanut butter, sesame tahini), Eastwind Nut Butters (peanut, cashew, tahini, almond), Eden Organic Apple Butter, Joyva Sesame Tahini, Maranata Roasted (pistachio butter, filbert butter, sunflower butter, almond butter), Maranata (sesame tahini, cashew butter, almond butter) Once Again Hazelnut Butter, Sahadi Sesame Butter, Santa Cruz Organic (apple apricot sauce, apple sauce), Westbrae Natural (raw sesame tahini, toasted tahini).

- Breads—French Meadow Bakery, Garden of Eatin (blue corn and corn tortillas), Lundberg Rice Cakes, Manna, New Pioneer Co-op (farm bread, olive farm, raisin pecan, sourdough, wheat).

- Canned beans—American Prairie, Bearitos Refried Fat Free, Eden, Shari's, Westbrae Natural Garbanzo.
- Salsas—Garden Valley Naturals, Muir Glen, New Bounty Organic, Parrot.
- Pasta sauces—Eden (spaghetti sauce, pizza-pasta sauce), Garden Valley Organic, Millina's Finest Organic, Muir Glen Organic.
- Pastas/noodles—Eden, Millina's Finest, Vita Spelt.
- Tofu/tempeh/soy/miso—American Pride Tofu, Earth Fire Products, Eden products, White Wave (organic wild rice tempeh, five grain tempeh, soy tempeh, sea veggie tempeh, organic tofu).
- Frozen foods—Cascadian Farms (organic broccoli, corn, plain vegetables, raspberries, blueberries, strawberries), Sno-Pac (organic vegetables).
- Teas—Alvita, Celestial Seasonings (except for its vitamin enriched teas), Choice Organic, Eden Great Eastern Sun, Long Life Organic, Maharishi Ayur-Veda (Vata, Pitta and Kapha Churnas and Teas, and Raja's Cup), Traditional Medicinals, Yogi Organic.
- Juices—Organic with no vitamins added: After the Fall (Vermont Harvest Moon, apple cider, grape juice), Crofters (guava, strawberry, papaya, raspberry, apricot, pink lemon-ade), Eden (organic apple, organic tomato, organic cherry), Kedem (100-percent-pure grape juice), Knudsen (cherry, grape, mango, pea, strawberry), Mountain Sun (organic strawberry, peach, blueberry, cranberry), Santa Cruz (ginger, apricot, cherry, raspberry, apple).
- Chips/snacks/candies—Eden, Little Bear Lite Organic Popcorn, Manischewitz Passover Matzos (tea matzos and whole wheat tea matzos), Reeds Crystallized Ginger, St. Claire Organic (winter mints, licorice sweets, cinnamon snaps, cherry sweets, lemon tarts, peppermints, cocoa sweets, ginger snaps), dried non-GE fruit (either unsweetened or approved non-GE sweetener), Westbrae Organic Potato Chips.

THE COUNCIL for Responsible Genetics and High Mowing Organic Seed Farm have started a project called the Safe Seed Initiative. The effort asks seed companies to sign a pledge not to use genetically engineered seeds. Below is a list of companies that have explicitly agreed not to use genetically engineered seeds. (See page 217 for a complete list of organic seed companies, some of which have signed this pledge. Even those who haven't are likely to be GE-free.)

Arkansas:
Horus Botanicals
   HCR Rt. 82, Box 29
   Salem, AR 72576

Arizona:
Native Seeds/SEARCH
   526 North 4th Avenue
   Tucson, AZ 85705
   Tel: 520–622–5561
   Fax: 520–622–5591
   Web site: www.nativeseeds.org

California:
Bountiful Gardens
   18001 Shafer Ranch Road
   Willits, CA 95490
   Tel: 707–459–6410
   Fax:707–459–1925
   E-mail: bountiful@sonic.net
   Web site: www.bountifulgardens.org

Environmental Seed Producers
  P.O. Box 2709
  Lompoc, CA 93438
  Tel: 805–735–8888
  Fax: 805–735–8798
  Web site: www.espseeds.com

Harmony Farm Supply and Nursery
  P.O. Box 460
  Graton, CA 95444
  Tel: 707–823–9125
  Fax: 707–823–1734
  E-mail: info@harmonyfarm.com
  Web site: www.harmonyfarm.com

KUSA Seed Research Foundation
  P.O. Box 761
  Ojai, CA 93024

Mountain Rose Herbs
  20818 High Street
  North San Juan, CA 95960
  Tel: 530–292–9138
  Fax: 510–217–4012
  Web site: www.mountainroseherbs.com

Natural Gardening Company
  P.O. Box 750776
  Petaluma, CA 94975-0776
  Tel: 707–766–9303
  Fax: 707–766–9747
  Web site: www.naturalgardening.com

Peaceful Valley Farm Supply
P.O. Box 2209
Grass Valley, CA 95945
Tel: 888–784–1722
Fax: 530–272–4769
E-mail: contact@groworganic.com
Web site: www.groworganic.com

Redwood City Seed Company
P.O. Box 361
Redwood City, CA 94064
Tel: 650–325–7333
Web site: www.ecoseeds.com

Renee's Garden
7359 West Zayante Road
Felton, CA 95018
Tel: 831–335–7228
Fax: 831–335–7227
Web site: www.reneesgarden.com

Santa Barbara Heirloom Nursery
P.O. Box 4235
Santa Barbara, CA 93140
Tel: 805–968–5444
Fax: 805–562–1248
E-mail: Heirloom@heirloom.com

Seed Dreams
P.O. Box 1476
Santa Cruz, CA 95061
Tel: 831–234–8668

Colorado:

Beauty Beyond Belief Wildflower Seeds
1730 So. College Avenue, #104
Fort Collins 80525
Tel: 970–221–3039

Sourcepoint Organic Seeds
1452 2900 Road
Hotchkiss, CO 81419
Tel: 970–250–0951

Sunnyland Seeds
P.O. Box 385
Paradox, CO 81429
Tel: 970–859–7248

Connecticut:

Butterbrooke Farm
78 Barry Road
Oxford, CT 06478
Tel: 203–888–2000

Comstock Ferre & Co.
263 Main Street
Wethersfield, CT 06109
Tel: 860–571–6950
Fax: 860–571–6595
Web site: www.comstockferre.com

John Scheepers Kitchen Garden Seeds
23 Tulip Drive
Bantam, CT 06750
Tel: 860–567–6086
Fax: 860–567–5323
Web site: www.kitchengardenseeds.com

New England Seed Company
  3580 Main Street, Bldg 10
  Hartford, CT 06120
  Tel: 800–783–7891 or 860–724–1240
  Fax: 860–724–1273
  E-mail: newenglsee@aol.com
  Web site: www.neseed.com

Select Seeds Company
  180 Stickney Hill Road
  Union, CT 06076
  Tel: 860–684–9310
  Fax: 860–684–9224
  E-mail: info@selectseeds.com
  Web site: www.selectseeds.com

Florida:

E.O.N.S., Inc.
  P.O. Box 4604
  Hallandale, FL 33008
  Tel: 954–455–0229
  Fax: 954–458–5976
  Web site: www.eonseed.com

Florida Mycology Research Center
  P.O. Box 18105
  Pensacola, FL 32523
  Tel: 850–327–4378
  Web site: www.mushroomsfmrc.com

The Pepper Gal
  P.O. Box 23006
  Ft. Lauderdale, FL 33307
  Tel: 954–537–5540
  Fax: 954–566–2208
  E-mail: peppergal@mindspring.com

Georgia:

Tanager Song Farm
P.O. Box 2143
Toccoa, GA 30577
Tel: 864–647–6434
E-mail: cindymcdee@aol.com
Web site: www.cindymcdee.com

Idaho:

High Altitude Gardens and Seeds Trust
4150 Black Oak Drive
Hailey, ID 83333
Tel: 208–788–4363
Fax: 208–788–3452
E-mail: mcdorman@seedsave.org

Illinois:

Borries Open Pollinated Seed Corn Farm
16293 E. 1400th Avenue
Teutopolis, IL 62467
Tel: 217–857–3377

Underwood Gardens
1414 Zimmerman Road
Woodstock, IL 60098
E-mail: info@underwoodgardens.com
Web site: www.underwoodgardens.com

Indiana:

E&R Seed
1356 East 200S
Monroe, IN 46772

Iowa:

Sand Hill Preservation Center
1878 230th Street
Calamus, IA 52729
Tel: 319–246–2299

Seed Savers Exchange
3076 North Winn Road
Decorah, IA 52101
Tel: 319–382–5990
Fax: 319–382–5872
Web site: www.seedsavers.org

Kansas:

Skyfire Garden Seeds
1313 23rd Road
Kanopolis, KS 67454
E-mail: seedsaver@myvine.com
Web site: www.grapevine.net/~mctaylor

Kentucky:

England's Orchard and Nursery
316 Kentucky Highway 2004
McKee, KY 40447
Tel: 606–965–2228
Fax: 606–965–2270
E-mail: nuttrees@prtcnet.org
Web site: www.nuttrees.net

Ferry Morse Seed Company
600 Stephen Beale Drive
P.O. Box 1620
Fulton, KY 42041
Tel: 800–626–3392
Fax: 502–472–0566

Shooting Star Nursery
   444 Bates Road
   Frankfort, KY 40601
   Tel: 502–223–1679
   Fax: 502–227–5700

Maine:
FedCo Seeds
   P.O. Box 520
   Waterville, ME 04903
   Tel: 207–873–7333
   Fax: 207–872–8317
   Web site: www.fedcoseeds.com

Johnny's Selected Seeds
   184 Foss Hill Road
   P.O. Box 2580
   Albion, ME 04910
   Tel: 207–437–9294
   Fax: 207–437–2165
   E-mail: info@johnnyseeds.com
   Web site: www.johnnyseeds.com

Maine Seed Saving Network
   P.O. Box 126
   Penobscot, ME 04476
   Tel: 207–362–0751

Old Stage Farm
   RR2 Box 377
   Lovell, ME 04051
   Tel: 207–925–1006

Wood Prairie Farm Organic Seed Potatoes
49 Kinney Road
Bridgewater, ME 04735
Tel: 800–829–9765
Fax: 800–300–6494
Web site: www.woodprarie.com

Maryland:
Silver Seed Greenhouses
P.O. Box 62
Bivalve, MD 21814
Tel: 410–873–2942
Fax: 410–873–2728
E-mail: ubuubok@dmv.com

Massachusetts:
Eastern Native Seed Conservancy
P.O. Box 451
Great Barrington, MA 01230
Tel: 413–229–8316
E-mail: natseeds@aol.com
Web site: www.enscseeds.org

Perennial Vegetable Seed Company
P.O. Box 608
Belchertown, MA 01007
Tel: 413–529–0678

Pioneer Valley Seed Collective
(Formerly Pioneer Valley Seed Savers)
888 Shelburne Falls Road
Conway, MA 01341
Tel: 413–369–4269
Fax: 413–369–4299

Minnesota:

Melissa's Seeds
P.O. Box 242
Hastings, MN 55033

Missouri:

Baker Creek Heirloom Seeds
2278 Baker Creek Road
Mansfield, MO 65704
Tel: 417–924–8917
Fax: 417–924–8917
E-mail: seeds@rareseeds.com
Web site: www.rareseeds.com

Barney's Ginseng Patch
433 SSE Highway B
Montgomery City, MO 63361
Tel: 573–564–2575

Elixir Farm
General Delivery
Brixey, MO 65618
Tel: 417–261–2393
Fax: 417–261–2355
E-mail: info@elixirfarm.com
Web site: www.elixirfarm.com

Green Thumb Seeds
17011 West 280th Street
Bethany, MO 64424

Jon's Heirloom Plants
P.O. Box 54
Mansfield, MO 65704
E-mail: jon@jonsplants.com

Morgan County Wholesale
  18761 Kelsay Road
  Barnett, MO 65011
  Tel: 573–378–2655

Montana:
Swan View Farm LLC
  345 Rocky Woods Lane
  Bigfork, MT 59911–6324
  Tel: 888–845–7623
  Fax: 406–837–2817
  Web site: www.thepowerofgarlic.com

Nebraska:
The Fragrant Path
  Seeds for Fragrance
  P.O. Box 328
  Ft. Calhoun, NE 68023

New Jersey:
Garden State Heirloom Seed Society
  P.O. Box 15
  Delaware, NJ 07833
  Tel: 908–475–4861
  E-mail: njheirloom@earthlink.net
  Web site: www.gshss.com

New Mexico:
Plants of the Southwest
  3095 Aqua Fria Road
  Santa Fe, NM 87507
  Tel: 505–438–8888
  Fax: 505–438–8800
  Web site: www.plantsofthesouthwest.com

Seeds of Change
P.O. Box 15700
Santa Fe, NM 87592
Tel: 888–762–7333
E-mail: gardener@seedsofchange.com
Web site: www.seedsofchange.com

North Carolina:
Boone's Native Seed Company
P.O. Box 10363
Raleigh, NC 27605

Christopher Weeks Peppers
P.O. Box 3207
Kill Devil Hills, NC 27948
E-mail: peppers@pinn.net

Ohio:
Companion Plants, Inc.
7247 N. Coolville Ridge
Athens, OH 45701
Tel: 740–592–4643
Fax: 740–593–3092
E-mail: complants@frognet.net
Web site: www.companionplants.com

Mellinger's
2310 W. South Range Road
North Lima, OH 44452
Tel: 330–549–9861
Fax: 330–549–3716
E-mail: mellgarden@mellingers.com
Web site: www.mellingers.com

Oregon:

Goodwin Creek Gardens
P.O. Box 83
Williams, OR 97544
Tel: 800–846–7359
Fax: 541–846–7357
Web site: www.goodwincreekgardens.com

Horizon Herbs
P.O. Box 69
Williams, OR 97544
Tel: 541–846–6704
Fax: 541–846–6233
E-mail: herbseed@chatlink.com

Nichol's Garden Nursery
1190 Old Salem Road, NE
Albany, OR 97321
Tel: 541–928–9280 or 800–422–3985
Fax: 541–967–8406
E-mail: nichols@gardennursery.com
Web site: www.nicholsgardennursery.com

Peters Seed and Research
P.O. Box 1472
Myrtle Creek, OR 97457
Tel: 541–874–2615
Fax: 541–874–3462
E-mail: psr@pioneer-net.com

Sow Organic Seed
P.O. Box 527
1130 Tetherow Road
Williams, OR 97544
Web site: www.organicseed.com

Territorial Seed Company
  P.O. Box 158
  Cottage Grove, OR 97424
  Tel: 541–942–9547
  Fax: 541–942–9881
  E-mail: tsc@ordata.com
  Web site: www.territorial-seed.com

Thyme Garden—Herb Seed Company
  20546 Alsea Highway
  Alsea, OR 97324
  Tel & Fax: 541–487–8671
  E-mail: herbs@thymegarden.com
  Web site: www.thymegarden.com

Victory Seed Company
  P.O. Box 192
  Molalla, OR 97038
  Tel/Fax: 503–829–3126
  E-mail: safeseed@victoryseeds.com
  Web site: www.victoryseeds.com

Wild Garden Seed and Shoulder to Shoulder Farm
  P.O. Box 1509
  Philomath, OR 97370
  Tel: 541–929–4068

Pennsylvania:
Bethlehem Seed Company
  P.O. Box 1351
  Bethlehem, PA 18018
  Tel: 610–954–5443

Landis Valley Museum
  Heirloom Seed Project
  2451 Kissel Hill Road
  Lancaster, PA 17601
  Tel: 717–569–0401 ext: 202
  Fax: 717–560–2147
  Web site: landisvalleymuseum.org

Heirloom Seeds
  P.O. Box 245
  West Elizabeth, PA 15088
  Tel/Fax: 412–384–0852
  E-mail: mail@heirloomseeds.com
  Web site: www.heirloomseeds.com

South Carolina:
Seeds for the South
  410 Whaley Pond Road
  Graniteville, SC 29829
  Tel: 803–232–1119
  E-mail: seedsout@mindspring.com

Texas:
The Herb Cottage
  442 CR 233
  Hallettsville, TX 77964-4048
  Tel & Fax: 979–562–2153
  E-mail: herbs@theherbcottage.com
  Web site: www.theherbcottage.com

Vermont:
The Cook's Garden
  P.O. Box 535
  Londonderry, VT 05148
  Tel: 800–457–9703
  Fax: 802–824–9556

E-mail: catalog@cooksgarden.com
Web site: www.cooksgarden.com

Dirt Works
  6 Dog Team Road
  New Haven, VT 05472
  Tel: 802–453–5373
  E-mail: dirtworks@globalnetisp.net
  Web site: www.dirtworks.net

High Mowing Seeds
  813 Brook Rd
  Wolcott, VT 05680
  Tel: 802–888–1800
  Fax: 802–888–8446
  Web site: www.highmowingseeds.com

Ladybug Herbs of Vermont
  943 Richard Woolcutt Road
  Wolcott, VT 05680
  Tel/Fax: 802–888–5940
  E-mail: vtherbs@pover.net
  Web site: www.ladybugherbsofvermont.com

North Wind Organic Seeds
  (Formerly Arethusa Seed Farm)
  P.O. Box 175
  Bakersfield, VT 05441
  Tel/Fax: 802–827–6580

Vermont Organic Seeds
  12 Dudley Street
  Randolph VT 05060
  E-mail: cyczapla@yahoo.com
  Web site: www.sover.net/~subzero/seedlist.html

Weed Farm Herbs
  613 Quaker Street
  Lincoln, VT 05443
  Tel: 802–453–7395
  E-mail: weedfarm@gmavt.net

Virginia:

Garden Medicinals and Culinaries
  P.O. Box 320
  Earlysville, VA 22936
  Tel: 804–964–9113
  Fax: 804–973–8717
  Web site: www.gardenmedicinals.com

Thomas Jefferson Center for Historic Plants
  P.O. Box 316, Monticello
  Charlottesville, VA 22902
  Tel: 804–984–9821
  Fax: 804–984–0358
  Web site: www.monticello.org/shop

Washington:

Abundant Life Seed Foundation
  P.O. Box 772
  Port Townsend, WA 98368
  Tel: 360–385–5660
  Fax: 360–385–7455
  E-mail: abundant@olypen.com
  Web site: abundantlifeseed.com

Filaree Farm
  182 Conconully Hwy.
  Okanogan, WA 98840
  Tel: 509–422–6940
  E-mail: filaree@northcascades.com
  Web site: www.filareefarm.com

Frosty Hollow Ecological Restoration
   Box 53
   Langley, WA 98260
   Tel: 360–579–2332
   Fax: 360–579–4080
   E-mail: wean@whidbey.net

Fungi Perfecti
   P.O. Box 7634
   Olympia, WA 98507
   Tel: 360–426–9292
   Fax: 360–426–9377

Garlicsmiths
   967 Mingo Mountain Road
   Kettle Falls, WA 99141
   Tel: 509–738–4470

Irish Eyes-Garden City Seeds
   P.O. Box 307
   Thorpe, WA 98946
   Tel: 509–964–7000
   Fax: 800–964–9210
   E-mail: potatoes@irish-eyes.com
   Web site: www.irish-eyes.com

Wisconsin:
Island Seed and Supply
   19370 Highway G
   Mineral Point, WI 53565
   Tel: 608–776–3414

Superior Organic Grains, Ltd
   N7076
   Seymour, WI 54165

Canada:

Alberta Nurseries and Seeds, Ltd.
P.O. Box 20
Bowden, Alberta T0M 0K0
Tel: 403–224–3544
Fax: 403–224–2455

Aurora
4492 Phillps Road
Creston, British Columbia V0B1G2
Tel: 250–428–4404
E-mail: aurora@kootenay.com
Web site: www.kootenay.com/~aurora

Ecogenesis, Inc.
#88–2273 Yonge Street
Toronto, Ontario M4P 2C6
Tel: 416–485–8333

Eternal Seed
657 Pritchard Road
Farrellton, Quebec J0X 1T0
Tel: 819–827–2795
E-mail: edecas@travel-net.com

Fish Lake Garlic Man
RR2
Demorestville, Ontario K0K 1WO
Tel: 613–476–8030

Florabunda Seeds
P.O. Box 3
Indian River, Ontario K0L 2B0
Tel: 705–295–6440
Fax: 705–295–4035
E-mail: contact@florabundaseeds.com
Web site: www.florabundaseeds.com

Mapple Farm
129 Beech Hill Road
Weldon, New Brunswick E0A 1X0
Tel: 506–734–3361

Prairie Garden Seeds
P.O. Box 118
Cochin, Saskatchewan S0M 0L0
Tel: 306–386–2737
E-mail: prairie.seeds@sk.sympatico.ca

Richter's Herbs
357 Hwy 47
Goodwood, Ontario L0C 1A0
Tel: 905–640–6677
Fax: 905–640–6641
E-mail: orderdesk@richters.com
Web site: www.richters.com

Salt Spring Seeds
P.O. Box 444, Ganges
Salt Spring Island, British Columbia V8K 2W1
Tel: 250–537–5269
Web site: www.saltspring.com/ssseeds

Terra Edibles
P.O. Box 164
Foxboro, Ontario K0K 2B0
Tel: 613–968–8238
Fax: 613–968–6369

West Coast Seeds Ltd.
3925 64 Street, RR 1,
Delta, British Columbia V4K 3N2
Tel: 604–952–8820
Fax: 604–952–8828
E-mail: info@westcoastseeds.com
Web site: www.westcoastseeds.com

MEAT AND POULTRY

WHILE FOOD derived from genetically engineered animals is not currently being sold in supermarkets—except for dairy products coming from diary cows injected with the genetically engineered milk hormone rBGH—experimental transgenic pigs, cattle, and fish are expected to be commercialized soon. But the real concern right now is with animal feed. Up to 80 percent of genetically engineered grain is being utilized for animal feed.[8]

In response to public concerns about the safety of meat, eggs, and poultry in general, a burgeoning market is evolving in GE-free, organic/free-range/no hormone meat. In January 1999, for the first time, the U.S. Department of Agriculture allowed meat to be labeled as organic. The rule allows organic certification agencies to certify as "organic" meat produced by farmers that do not use pesticide-treated feed, growth hormones, or antibiotics. Additionally, current organic rules require that meat and poultry are raised on organic feed, without the use of antibiotics or growth hormones, that the animals have access to fresh water and pasture, and that there is a manure-management plan.

Organic meat is a rapidly growing segment of the organic market. And the growing opposition to GE in the U.S. will undoubtedly fuel an even greater demand for organic meat labeled as GE-free. Federal regulations on organic standards, that came into force in October 2002, require all certified organic animals to be fed 100 percent organic feed—thereby excluding all GE-derived feed.

A recent survey done by Greenpeace in the United Kingdom found that major food retailers are rushing to source meat, eggs, and dairy products from non-GE-fed animals to counter widespread customer concern. Tesco, the largest food retailer in the UK, has already written to major international animal feed suppliers Cargill and Archer Daniel Midlands, informing them of their intention to eliminate genetically engineered ingredients in animal feed.[9]

Besides your local co-op or supermarket there are numerous other companies selling organic meat that you can contact directly. See chapter 10 for a list of companies selling organic meat and poultry. The best resource for sustainably raised meat, poultry, and fish on the Web is the Institute for Agriculture and Trade Policy's Eat Well Guide: www.eatwellguide.org.

WHO OFFERS RBGH-FREE MILK?

SINCE THE recombinant Bovine Growth Hormone (rBGH) was introduced onto the market in 1994, a limited percentage of the U.S. milk supply has come from cows injected with the hormone. Since the milk of many different cows is routinely comingled in bulk tanks at most of the nation's dairies, this means that the majority of non-organic dairy products probably contain at least trace levels of rBGH. While the USDA reported in 2002 that 22 percent of the nation's dairy cows are injected with rBGH, critics of the drug believe the actual figure is more like 10 percent. In response to rBGH's introduction into the milk business, several hundred companies now require written affidavits from their milk suppliers that no rBGH was injected into the cows, and label the milk as rBGH-free. Approximately 10 percent of fluid milk in the U.S. is now labeled rBGH-free.

That percentage of cows injected with rBGH is expected to be cut in half in 2004. In January 2004, Monsanto sent a letter to farmers saying that they would only allocate 50 percent of the rBGH they had in the past, because a factory producing the hormone had failed a FDA inspection for quality control.[10]

Others have capitalized on the growing market niche of organic milk, which is guaranteed to be GE-free since organic certification prohibits the use of rBGH. Since the introduction of rBGH, sales of organic milk have skyrocketed. For instance, sales grew from $16 million in 1996, to $31 million in 1997.[11]

Ben & Jerry's Homemade Inc. takes steps to ensure that the milk in its ice cream does not come from cows injected with recombinant Bovine Growth Hormone. The company is also making sure that brownies and other ingredients are not made from genetically engineered ingredients.

All dairy products made from sheep or goat's milk are rBGH-free because the drug is not used with these animals. Recombinant Bovine Growth Hormone is not approved for use in Canada, the European Union, New Zealand, and Australia. Cheeses and other dairy products from any of these countries are rBGH-free.

Below is a partial list, compiled by the Organic Consumers Association, of milk and dairy companies that have pledged that their milk does not come from cows injected with the Bovine Growth Hormone. The first section lists companies with organic dairy products; the second section lists companies with rBGH-free (but not necessarily organic) products. Those marked with "*" are small family farms.

RBGH-FREE (ORGANIC)

California

- Straus Family Creamery* (milk, butter, yogurt, cheese), Marshall, CA, 415–663–5464, www.strausmilk.com
  Available in California, Arizona, and New Mexico.
- Alta Dena Organics (cheese), City of Industry, CA, 800–535–1369
  Available nationwide.

Colorado

- Horizon Organic Dairy (milk, chocolate milk, cream, whipped cream, yogurt, cheese, butter, sour cream, cottage cheese, cream cheese), Boulder, CO, 888–494–3020
  Available nationwide.

Iowa

- Radiance Dairy* (milk, whipping cream, yogurt, and several cheeses), Fairfield, IA, 641–472–8554
  Available at Hy-Vee, Econo Foods, and Everybody's Whole Foods in the Fairfield area and at New Pioneer Co-op in Iowa City.

Maine

- Hart-to-Hart Farm* (cheese and licensed raw milk), Albion, ME, 207–437–2441
  Available at the farm and at farmers' markets throughout central Maine (call for locations).
- Nezinscot Farm* (cow's or goat's milk, cheese, butter), Turner, ME, 207–225–3231
  Available at their own store in Turner; cheese available by mail order.

Massachusetts

- Bart's Homemade (low-fat organic ice cream), Greenfield, MA, 413–774–7438

  Available in Massachusetts, New Hampshire, Connecticut, and at their own store in Greenfield.

- Brookside Farm* (milk and cream), Westminster, MA, 978–874–2695

  Available in Massachusetts.

Missouri

- Morningland Dairy Cheese*, Mountain View, MO, 417–469–3817

  Available nationwide and by mail order.

Montana

- Lifeline Farms* (cheese), Victor, MT

  Available on the West Coast.

  For store locations, call Mountain Peoples, 800–679–8735, www.csf.Colorado.edu/co-op/mountain.html.

New Hampshire

- Stonyfield Farms (organic line) (yogurt and ice cream), Londonderry, NH, 603–437–4040

  Available nationwide.

New York

- Hawthorne Valley Farm* (cheese, yogurt and quark cheese), Ghent, NY, 518–672–7500

  Available on the East Coast. Raw milk and cheese also available at their own local store and at the Union Square Farmers' Market in New York City.

- Butternut Farms* (cheese), NY, 607–783–2392, www.butternutfarms.com

  Available in the Northeast and by mail order.

- Natural by Nature (cheese, cream, buttermilk, eggnog, ice cream, butter, yogurt, cream cheese, milk, pudding), Sunnydale Farms, Brooklyn, NY, 718–257–7600
  Available on the East Coast and in the Midwest.

Oregon

- Echo Spring Dairy (organic line) (milk, sour cream, cottage cheese), Eugene, OR, 541–753–7331
  Available in Idaho, Oregon, and northern California.

Pennsylvania

- Kimberton Hills Farm* (licensed raw milk), Kimberton, PA, 610–935–0314
  Available at Kimberton Whole Foods store (610–935–1444), and at the farm.
- Seven Stars Farm* (yogurt), Phoenixville, PA 610–935–1949
  Available in the East and Midwest.

Vermont

- Animal Farm Butter (organic butter), Orwell, VT, 802–623–6599, www.animalfarmvt.com/
  Available at Middlebury Natural Food Coop in Middlebury.
- Butterworks Farm* (yogurt, cream, cheese, cottage cheese), Westfield, VT, 802–744–6855
  Available in the Northeast and at the farm; cheese also available by mail order.
- Organic Cow of Vermont (milk, chocolate milk, sour cream, cottage cheese, butter, cream, eggnog), Chelsea, VT, 800–769–9693
  Available on the East Coast.

- Greenbank Farms Cheese (organic line), Stonefelt Cheese Co., Preston, WA, 425–222–5500
    Available on the West Coast, in the northwest, and at their own store in Preston.
- Cascadian Farm (frozen yogurt, ice cream), Sedro-Wooley, WA, 800–624–4123
    Available nationwide.

Wisconsin
- Ranovael Organic Dairy* (cheese, butter), DePere, WI, 920–336–2820
    Cheese available by mail order, both products available at their own store in DePere.
- Cedar Grove Organic Cheese, Plain, WI, 608–546–5284, www.cedargrovecheese.com
    Available in the upper Midwest, at their own store in Plain, and by mail order (800) 200–6020).
- Organic Valley* (milk, cheese, butter, cream cheese, cottage cheese, sour cream, cream, powdered milk), La Farge, WI, 608–625–2600, www.organicvalley.com
    Available nationwide.
- Wisconsin Organics* (milk, cheese, butter), Bonduel, WI, 715–758–2280
    Available nationwide and at their own retail store in Bonduel.

RBGH-FREE (BUT NOT ORGANIC) BRANDS

California
- Clover Stornetta Farms (milk, cheese, sour cream, yogurt), Petaluma, CA, 800–237–3315, www.clo-the-cow.com
    Available in northern California.

- Joseph Farms Cheese, Joseph Gallo, Atwater, CA, 209–394–7984, www.josephfarms.com
  Available in the Northwest, Southwest, South, and Hawaii.
- Alta Dena (milk, buttermilk, chocolate milk, eggnog, cream, sour cream, yogurt, natural select butter, ice cream, cottage cheese, and all cheeses except for cream cheese), City of Industry, CA, 800–MILK123
  Available nationwide.
- Brown Cow Farm (yogurt and milk), Antioch, CA, 925–757–9209, www.wholemilkyogurt.com
  Available nationwide.
- Lifetime Dairy (cheese), Lifeline Food Co., Seaside, CA, 831–899–5040, www.lifetimefatfree.com
  Available nationwide.
- Berkeley Farms (full line of dairy products), Hayward, CA, 510–265–8600, www.berkeleyfarms.com
  Available in northern California.

Connecticut
- Rustling Winds Creamery (cheese, milk but bring your own container), Falls Village, CT, 860–824–7084
  Available at their farm store; cheese available by mail order.
- Calabro Cheese Corp., East Haven, CT, 203–469–1311, www.calabrocheese.com
  Available on the East and West Coasts and in Ohio.

Florida
- Golden Fleece Dairy* (milk), Lecanto, FL, 352–628–2688
  Available in Florida.

Illinois

- Oberweiss Dairy (milk and ice cream), Aurora, IL, 630–897–6600

  Available in Illinois.

Louisiana

- Mauthe's Dairy* (whole milk, skim milk, creole cream cheese), Folsom, LA, 985–796–5058

  www.mauthescreolecreamcheese.com/index.htm

  Available in New Orleans area, Cresent City Farmers Markets, Covington Farmers Markets and online.

Maine

- Kate's Homemade Butter, Old Orchard Beach, ME, 207–934–5134

  Available nationwide.

Massachusetts

- Balance Rock Farm (milk), Berlin, MA, 978–838–2024

  Available at their farm store in Berlin.

- Brigham's Ice Cream, Arlington, MA, 800–BRIGHAMS, www.brighams.com

  Available in the Northeast.

- Crescent Creamery (milk), Pittsfield, MA, 800–221–6455

  Available in the Northeast.

- Dorchester Ice Cream, Boston, MA, 617–282–9600

  Available in the Northeast.

- Great Hill Dairy (cheese), Marion, MA, 508–748–2208, www.greathillblue.com

  Available by mail order or nationwide at gourmet stores.

Michigan

- Crooked Creek Farm Dairy (milk, ice cream), Romeo, MI, 810–752–6095

  Available at Farm Dairy store and at select stores in southeast Michigan.

- Jilbert's Dairy (milk, ice cream), Marquette, MI, 906–225–1363

  Available in Michigan's upper peninsula through Wisconsin border.
- Pollard Dairy (milk, chocolate milk, whipped cream), Norway, MI, 906–563–8815

  Available in Michigan's upper peninsula, northeastern Wisconsin.

Minnesota

- Cedar Summit* (milk, butter, dips, ice cream, hard cheeses and yogurt), New Prague, MN 952–758–6886

  www.cedarsummit.com

  Available in Twin Cities area and in Northfield, New Prague, and St. Peter, MN.
- Sonny's Ice Cream (ice cream), Minneapolis, MN, 612–822–8189

  Available in the Twin Cities metro area, the Chicago area, and by phone orders. All dairy ingredients are from the Pride of Main Street Dairy.
- Polka Dot Dairy (milk, half-and-half, whole cream, buttermilk), Hastings, MN, 651–437–9023

  Available at all Tom Thumb stores in Minnesota and Wisconsin.
- Valley View Farms (milk, half-and-half, whole cream, buttermilk), Hastings, MN, 651–437–9414

  Available in eastern Minnesota and western Wisconsin.
- Pride of Main Street (milk, ice cream), Sauk Centre, MN, 320–351–8300

  Available only in Minnesota.
- Schroder Simply Right (milk), Mapelwood, MN, 651–487–1471

  Available in Minnesota and western Wisconsin. Bottles rBGH-free milk for SuperAmerica that is sold only in returnable gallons under the SuperAmerica label.

- Kemp's Select (milk), Kemp's Marigold Foods, Minneapolis, MN, 800–726–6455

  Available in Minnesota and Eau Clarie, Wisconsin.
- Land O Lakes' Original (milk) Arden Hills, MN 651–481–2222

  Available nationwide.

New Hampshire
- Hatchland Dairy* (milk, chocolate milk, egg nog, cream), N. Haverhill, NH, 603–787–2388

  Available in New Hampshire and Vermont.
- McNamara Dairy* (milk, chocolate milk, eggnog, cream), West Lebanon, NH, 603–298–6666

  Available in New Hampshire and Vermont.
- Stonyfield Farms (yogurt, frozen yogurt, ice cream), Londonderry, NH, 603–437–5050, www.stonyfield.com

  Available nationwide.

New Jersey
- Farmland Dairies (milk, chocolate milk, cream), Wallington, NJ, 1–800–327–9522

  Available on the East Coast.
- Biazzo Dairy Products (cheese), Riverfield, NJ, 201–941–6800

  Available nationwide.

New York
- Derle Farms (milk with "no rBST" label only), Brooklyn, NY, 718–257–2040

  Available in New York and New Jersey.
- Egg Farm Dairy (butter, cheese, ice cream, cream), Peekskill, NY, 800–CREAMERY

  Available at their local retail store, by mail order, and nationwide at gourmet food stores.

Pennsylvania

- Erivan Dairy Yogurt*, Oreland, PA, 215–887–2009
  Available on the East Coast and in the Midwest.

Tennessee

- Cruze Farm Dairy* (churned buttermilk, unhomogenized whole milk, ice cream available seasonally), Knoxville, TN, 865–525–6966
  Available in Knoxville, Sevierville, and Maryville, Tennessee.

Texas

- Promised Land Dairy (milk) Floresville, TX, 210–533–9151, www.promisedlanddairy.com
  Available in Texas, Arkansas, Oklahoma, Louisiana, Kansas, and Missouri.

Utah

- Brown's Dairy Summit Valley (full line of fluid milk, including whipping cream, half-and-half and chocolate milk) Coalville, UT, 435–336–5952 or 801–355–6079, www.breedernet.com/ads/brown.htm
  Available in Wild Oats and Good Earth Markets in Salt Lake City, and Winegars Markets, Dicks Markets, Albertsons, Smith Stores in Davis County.
- Winder Dairy (full line of fluid milk), West Valley City, UT, 801–969–3401, www.winderdairy.com
  Available by home delivery in all of Utah.

Vermont

- Thomas Dairy (milk, cream, eggnog, chocolate milk, butter, sour cream, yogurt, buttermilk), Rutland, VT, 802–773–6788
  Available in central Vermont.
- Monument Farms* (milk, cottage cheese, buttermilk, cream), Middlebury, VT, 802–545–2119

Available in Vermont and at their own store in Weybridge, Vermont.

- Booth Brothers Dairy (milk, cream, chocolate milk, egg nog), Barre, VT, 802–476–6605

    Available in Vermont and New Hampshire.

- Orb Weaver Farm* (cheese), New Haven, VT, 802–877–3755

    Available in Vermont, by mail order, at the farm, and at Murray's Cheese Shop in New York City.

- Vermont Family Farms* (milk), Vermont Milk Producers, Whiting, VT, 802–897–2769

    Available in Vermont, New Hampshire, Massachusetts, and upstate New York.

- Wilcox Dairy (milk, ice cream), Manchester, VT, 800–262–1223

    Available in Vermont, New Hampshire, Massachusetts, and in upstate New York.

- Blythedale Farm Cheese*, Corinth, VT, 802-439-6575

    Available in the Northeast.

- Sugarbush Farm* (cheese), Woodstock, VT, 800–281–1757

    Available in the Northeast and by mail order.

- Ben & Jerry's Ice Cream, S. Burlington, VT, 802-846-1500, www.benjerry.com/ca/

    Available nationwide.

- Franklin County Cheese, Enosburg Falls, VT, 802–933–4338, www.franklinfoods.com

    Available nationwide.

- Crowley Cheese of Vermont, Healdville, VT, 802–259–2210, www.newenglandcheese.com/companies/crowley.html

    Available nationwide and by mail order.

- Grafton Village Cheese, Grafton, VT, 800–472–3866, 802–843–2221, www.graftonvillagecheese.com

    Available nationwide and by mail order.

- Shelburne Farms Farmhouse Cheddar Cheese*, Shelburne, VT, 802–985–8686

Available nationwide, by mail order, and at their own farm store.

Virginia
- Shenville Creamery (entire line of products—yogurt, ice cream, fluid milk, fresh cheeses, dips), Timberville, VA, 1–877–600–7440, www.shenville.com/pages/351204/
  Available in Richmond and northern Virginia at most Kroger stores.

Washington
- Smith Brothers Dairy (milk), Kent, WA, 206–682–7633 www.smithbrothersfarms.com
  Available in Washington.
- Vitamilk Inc. (full line of dairy products), Seattle, WA, 206–524–7070
  Available in Washington.
- Darigold Inc. (full line of dairy products), Seattle, WA, 206–284–7220
  Available in Washington, Idaho, Alaska, and Montana.

Wisconsin
- Chippewa Valley Cheese, Osseo, WI, 715–597–2366, www.chippewavalleycheese.com
  Available in Wisconsin, Minnesota, North Dakota, Arkansas, and by mail order from their Web site.
- Family Farms Defenders* (cheese), Madison, WI, 608–260–0900
  Available in Madison, Wisconsin, and nationwide by mail order.
- Cedar Grove's Family Farmer Cheeses*, Plain, WI, 608–546–5284, www.execpc.com/~cgcheese/
  Available in the upper Midwest, at their own store in Plain, and by mail order (800–200–6020).
- Westby Cooperative Creamery* (cottage cheese, sour cream,

french onion dip, butter, cheese), Westby, WI, 800-492-9282, www.westbycreamery.com

Available in Wisconsin, Minnesota, Iowa, and Illinois and at their own store in Westby; cheese available by mail order.

- North Farm Cooperative* (cheese), Madison, WI, 800–236–5880, 608–241–2667, www.northfarm-coop.com

Available nationwide and by mail order.

- Salemville Cheese, North Farm Cooperative, Madison, WI, 800–236–5880

Available nationwide and by mail order.

FINDING GE-FREE PET FOOD

IAMS CO., the Ohio-based pet-food manufacturer, recently told its grain suppliers it would no longer accept genetically engineered corn for use in its premium dog and cat chows unless the corn varieties were among the few approved by the European Union. Unfortunately, the same cannot be said for Alpo, which has tested positive for genetically engineered ingredients in its dog food, and Purina, which has said, "Because genetically modified grain and grain products constitute a significant portion of the supply of grain available throughout the U.S. for both human and pet foods, it is likely that our pet-food products contain genetically modified grain."[12]

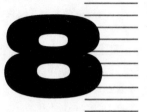

FOODS AND BRANDS YOU SHOULD
BUY AND WHERE YOU CAN FIND THEM

AS AN American consumer, you have been placed in a challenging situation if you want to avoid genetically engineered food. If there is no labeling, and conventional foods are mixed together with genetically engineered foods, how do you know what to avoid? Is it all simply luck of the draw? The situation leaves even the most careful consumer feeling vulnerable. Without question, it can be difficult to completely eliminate genetically engineered foods and ingredients from your diet. But, you can take several important steps that will dramatically reduce your exposure to genetically engineered food. By doing so, you will be supporting the type of farming that is decidedly against genetic engineering.

In order to buy GE-free foods, you'll have to play very close attention to where your food comes from, how it is produced, and who is producing it. You need to arm yourself with the best information available in order to make smart choices in the marketplace.

FIRST LINE OF DEFENSE—GO ORGANIC!

FIFTEEN YEARS ago, it was hard to find organic food in the marketplace. Organic food was considered an inconsequential segment of the food industry, to be found mostly in small co-ops, with little selection and expensive prices. But all that has changed. A 1999 Food Marketing Institute study found that organic and natural foods are available at approximately 73 percent of grocery stores and supermarkets. And the increase in accessibility is being driven by consumer demand. The FMI study also found that more than 50 percent of consumers seek out products labeled "organic," and 63 percent look for products labeled "natural."[1]

The organic food industry is the fastest growing sector of the food industry. Since 1989, it has grown 20–25 percent a year and is now estimated at over $13 billion a year in sales in North America. According to Datamonitor, the U.S. organic market is projected to reach a value of $30.7 billion by 2007, with a five-year compound annual growth rate of 21.4 percent between 2002 and 2007, compared to a 21.2 percent rate between 1997 and 2002.

In 2001, there were an estimated 7,800 U.S. farmers certified organic (with an estimated 1.3 million acres of certified organic cropland), according to the Organic Farming Research Foundation. When numbers are updated in 2004, there are expected to be around 10,000 organic farmers. The number of organic farmers is increasing by 12 percent a year, according to the USDA. These farms help to make organic food available at 400 co-ops, hundreds of farmers' markets, buying clubs, and even mainstream supermarkets. Organic products are now available in nearly 20,000 natural-food stores and 73 percent of conventional grocery stores, and account for approximately 1–2 percent of total food sales in the U.S.[2]

And in the summer of 2003, Whole Foods Market became the nation's first "Certified Organic" grocer, meaning retail operations have been certified organic by Quality Assurance International (QAI), a federally recognized independent third-party certification organization.

Organic agriculture is growing globally. Organic farming is practiced in approximately 100 countries throughout the world, with more than 24 million hectares (59 million acres) now under organic management. Australia leads with approximately 10 million hectares (24.6 million acres), followed by Argentina, with approximately 3 million hectares (7.4 million acres); both have extensive grazing land. Latin America has approximately 5.8 million hectares (14.3 million acres) under organic management, Europe has more than 5.5 million hectares (13.5 million acres), and North America has nearly 1.5 million hectares (3.7 million acres).[3]

The growth of the organic industry has been driven almost entirely by consumers and organic farmers—with almost no help from the government. The Organic Farm Research Foundation found in 2003 that, overall, organic research occupies only 1,160 acres (0.13 percent) of the 885,862 available research acres in the national land grant system.

There is good reason to believe that a major contributor to the organic industry's recent growth is the introduction of GE foods. "Organics have benefited, in the short run anyway, from GMOs because the only way to verify that you're not eating genetically modified organisms is to buy organic foods," says Karen Klonsky, an economist in the Department of Agricultural and Resource Economics at the University of California, Davis.[4]

The attraction to organic food is simple. Organic food is grown in a natural, environmentally safe manner without the use of synthetic pesticides, herbicides, or fertilizers. Instead, farmers rely on traditional farming methods that have been utilized for centuries—including crop rotation, the use of beneficial insects, composted manure as fertilizer—and a lot of hard work. Organic farming follows a philosophy of working with nature instead of working against it.

An added benefit of eating organic food is that it just might be more nutritious than conventional food. Although research on this issue is only just beginning in earnest, University of Copenhagen researchers have found that organic food contains more secondary metabolites than conventionally grown plants. Secondary metabolites are substances that form part of the plants' immune systems, and that also help to fight cancer in humans. Those same studies indicate that organic crops have measurably higher levels of vitamins.[5] Organically or sustainably grown berries and corn contain up to 58 percent more polyphenolics, natural antioxidants that are a natural defense for plants and may be good for our health, according to researchers at the University of California, Davis. The work suggests that pesticides and herbicides may actually reduce the production of polyphenolics by plants.[6] Other research has found that organically grown oranges contain up to 30 percent more vitamin C than those grown conventionally,[7] and that organic vegetable soups contain almost six times as much salicylic acid (which combats hardening of the arteries) as non-organic soups.[8] Fruits and veggies grown organically show significantly higher levels of cancer-fighting antioxidants than conventionally grown foods, according to a study of corn, strawberries, and marionberries.[9]

This new evidence on the nutritional value of organic food appears in stark contrast to the apparent nutrient declines on conventional food. In an analysis of USDA nutrient data from 1975 to 1997, the Kushi Institute of Becket, Massachusetts, found that the average calcium levels in twelve fresh vegetables declined 27 percent, iron levels dropped 37 percent, vitamin A levels 21 percent, and vitamin C levels 30 percent. A similar analysis of British nutrient data from 1930 to 1980 published in the British Food Journal found that in 20 vegetables, the average calcium content had declined 19 percent, iron 22 percent, and potassium 14 percent.[10]

And most importantly for the purposes of this book, organic

food production as enforced by the USDA certification system forbids the use of genetically engineered foods. USDA rules also explicitly forbid the use of genetically engineered ingredients in organic food production. However, it should be pointed out that there are still small possibilities that organic food could become contaminated with genetically engineered material. Processed or packaged organic foods can include up to 5 percent of non-organic ingredients. Those ingredients could be genetically engineered if the company has not ensured that its sources are not using genetically engineered crops. More and more organic companies are now taking steps to ensure that 100 percent of their ingredient sources are not genetically engineered.

In addition, organic fields are under constant threat from genetic contamination or drift from neighboring farms. There are the real-world events like the Terra Prima case detailed in chapter 2. In addition, a major organic farm in Britain was forced to decertify as organic after genetically engineered material drifted onto the farm. The Biotechnology Unit at the University of Glamorgan in the United Kingdom reported in February 2004 that eight of 25 food products labeled GE-free or organic contained levels of GE soy.

There is now a scientific consensus that genetically engineered material simply cannot be contained. The National Academy of Sciences issued a report in January 2004 that found that while there are many techniques being developed to prevent genetically engineered organisms or their genes from escaping into the wild, most techniques are still in early development and none appear to be completely effective.[11]

To combat this potential problem, more and more organic- and natural-food companies are having their sources and food tested to check for cases of drift. A Organic Research Foundation 2003 survey found that 17 percent companies surveyed have had GMO testing conducted on some portion of their organic farm seed, inputs, or farm products. Eleven percent of those that had GMO testing conducted indicated that they received positive test results for GMO contamination on some portion of their organic seed, inputs, or farm products.

TOP 10 REASONS TO BUY ORGANIC

1. **Protect future generations.** The average child receives four times more exposure than an adult to at least eight widely used cancer-causing pesticides in food. The food choices you make now will impact your child's health in the future.

2. **Prevent soil erosion.** The Soil Conservation Service estimates that more than 3 billion tons of topsoil are eroded from United States croplands each year. That means soil is eroding seven times faster than it is being built up naturally.

   Soil is the foundation of the food chain in organic farming. But in conventional farming the soil is used more as a medium for holding plants in a vertical position so they can be chemically fertilized. As a result, American farms are suffering from the worst soil erosion in history.

3. **Protect water quality.** Water makes up two-thirds of our body mass and covers three-fourths of the planet. Despite its importance, the Environmental Protection Agency (EPA) estimates pesticides—some cancer-causing—contaminate the groundwater in 38 states, polluting the primary source of drinking water for more than half the country's population.

4. **Save energy.** American farms have changed drastically in the last three generations, from family-based small businesses dependent on human energy to large-scale factory farms highly dependent on fossil fuels.

   Modern farming uses more petroleum than any other single industry, consuming 12 percent of the country's total energy supply. More energy is now used to produce synthetic fertilizers than to till, cultivate, and harvest all the crops in the United States.

   Organic farming is still mainly based on labor-intensive practices such as weeding by hand and using green manures and crop covers rather than synthetic fertilizers to build up soil. Organic produce also tends to travel fewer miles from field to table.

5. **Keep chemicals off your plate.** Many pesticides approved for use by the EPA were registered long before extensive research linking these chemicals to cancer and other diseases had been established. Now the EPA considers that 60 percent of all herbicides, 90 percent of all fungicides, and 30 percent of all insecticides are carcinogenic. A 1987 National Academy of Sciences report estimated that pesticides might cause an extra 1.4 million cancer cases among Americans over their lifetimes. The bottom line is that pesticides are poisons designed to kill living organisms, and can also be harmful to humans. In addition to cancer, pesticides are implicated in birth defects, nerve damage, and genetic mutation.

6. **Protect farm-worker health.** A National Cancer Institute study found that farmers exposed to herbicides had a six times greater risk than non-farmers of contracting cancer.

   In California, reported pesticide poisonings among farm workers have risen an average of 14 percent a year since 1973, and doubled between 1975 and 1985. Field workers suffer the highest rates of occupational illness in the state. Farm-worker health also is a serious problem in developing nations, where pesticide use can be poorly regulated. An estimated 1 million people are poisoned annually by pesticides.

7. **Help small farmers.** Although more and more large-scale farms are making the conversion to organic practices, most organic farms are small independently owned and operated family farms of less than 100 acres.

   It's estimated that the United States has lost more than 650,000 family farms in the past decade. Organic farming could be one of the few survival tactics left for family farms.

8. **Support a true economy.** Although organic foods might seem more expensive than conventional foods, conventional food prices do not reflect hidden costs borne by taxpayers, including billions of dollars annually in federal subsidies. Other hidden costs include pesticide regulation and testing, hazardous waste disposal and clean-up, and environmental damage.

   As health writer Gary Null has pointed out, if you add in the real environmental and social costs of irrigation to a head of lettuce, its price can range between $2 and $3.

9. **Promote biodiversity.** Mono-cropping is the practice of planting large plots of land with the same crop year after year. While this approach tripled

farm production between 1950 and 1970, the lack of natural diversity of plant life has left the soil lacking in natural minerals and nutrients. To replace the nutrients, chemical fertilizers are used often in increasing amounts.

Single crops are also much more susceptible to pests, making farmers more reliant on pesticides. Despite a tenfold increase in the use of pesticides between 1947 and 1974, crop losses due to insects have doubled—partly because some insects have become genetically resistant to certain pesticides.

10. **Taste better flavor.** There's a good reason why many chefs use organic foods in their recipes—they taste better! Organic farming starts with the nourishment of the soil, which eventually leads to the nourishment of the plant and, ultimately, our palates.

Source: Committee for Sustainable Agriculture

HOW DO YOU KNOW IT'S ORGANIC?

FINDING OUT whether a food is organic has become a lot simpler now that the new USDA national rules for organic, have been fully implemented. Organic food producers are currently required to be USDA-certified organic by official, independent agencies to make sure they are following procedures consistent with organic food production. Over 40 organic certification agencies nation-wide enforce the national standards. Eleven of the certification programs are state-run, while the rest are private or non-governmental certification agencies.

Under the new USDA organic rules, products labeled as "organic" must be composed of 95 percent organically produced ingredients. Processed products with 50–95 percent organic ingredients must use the phrase "made with organic ingredients." If a product is less than half organic, the organic items may be listed only in the ingredient list on the side panel.

Food is certified organic only when the certification agency is satisfied that the farm is meeting its standards for organic food production—i.e., not using toxic pesticides, genetically engineered crops or inputs, hormones, antibiotics, etc. If the food is not labeled "certified organic," then it has not been officially approved by these organic-certification bodies. However, thousands of small farmers in the U.S. do produce genuine organic products, even if they can't afford to pay certification fees.

Take notice that foods labeled as "natural" are not certified as organic. "Natural" simply means that a food or beverage has been produced without any artificial additives or preservatives. This is definitely a plus for consumers because this makes it easier to read the ingredients of natural products. However, just because a product is labeled "natural" does not mean it is GE-free. A growing number of natural food companies are taking steps to ensure that their ingredient sources are not genetically engineered, so look to see if the natural product has also labeled itself GE-free.

WHERE CAN YOU FIND ORGANIC FOOD? START AT THE SUPERMARKET

ORGANIC FOOD is no longer relegated strictly to the realm of neighborhood food co-ops, buying clubs, and farmers' markets. It can now be found in most major supermarkets, although you may have to look hard to find it—and the selection may not be adequate. Major supermarkets like Safeway, Krogers, Albertson's, Winn-Dixie, and Cub Foods now have organic sections, and are becoming more and more responsive to consumer demands for greater variety and quality. If the organic/natural food aisle isn't big enough, talk with the store manager, and make sure to keep buying organic. These supermarket chains track every purchase and are finely attuned to consumer trends.

In fact, the Minnesota-based Organic Alliance is working closely with a number of these mainstream supermarkets to make organic food products more available at some of the nation's largest supermarket chains—Kroger's, A&P, Wegmans, Publix, Byerly's, Lunds, Pratt Foods, King Soopers, and Food Emporium. An April

2000 promotion by the Organic Alliance targeted 500 supermarkets in cities in New York, New Jersey, Connecticut, Colorado, Minnesota, Wisconsin, Florida, Georgia, Illinois, Oklahoma, Oregon, California, and North and South Carolina.

But beyond the giant conventional supermarket chains, there are a growing number of specialty "organic and natural" food stores. The industry leaders are Whole Foods and Wild Oats. As we discussed in chapter 7, both Whole Foods and Wild Oats have made their own brand-name products GE–free. The Austin, Texas–based Whole Foods Market Inc. operates 148 stores (some under the name Fresh Fields) in North America and is America's first certified-organic grocer. Wild Oats, based in Boulder, Colorado, operates 101 stores.

JOIN A FOOD CO-OP

THE NUMBER and size of consumer food co-ops continues to grow in the U.S. There are now an estimated 350 co-ops located around the country, with over $500 million in annual sales—some co-ops now rival mainstream supermarket chains in terms of size and sales volume.[12] Food co-ops generally offer a full range of organic and natural food, and are set up to directly serve the needs and preferences of their members and customers. Co-ops are run democratically, and when you join, you become a part-owner. Food co-ops are non-profits, and often run at least partly on the power of volunteers. As a member of a co-op, you are usually entitled to certain discounts and even rebates at the end of the year. In the old days of co-ops, people qualified as members by volunteering time at the co-op. This concept is still alive at many U.S. co-ops, but most also offer the option of simply paying for membership. Generally, it is not necessary for you to become a formal member of a food co-op in order to shop at the store.

The best resource list for food co-ops is the National Co-op Directory, put out by the Co-op Network.

Co-op Network
P.O. Box 57
Randolph, VT 05060
802-234-9293

Another listing of co-ops on the Internet is the U.S. and Canadian Directory of Co-ops, which allows you to search by state to find a co-op near you: www.organicconsumers.org/store-search.htm

OWN A SHARE OF THE FARM— COMMUNITY-SUPPORTED AGRICULTURE

A GREAT way to get fresh organic produce and other food items— and support organic and small farms in your area—is by joining a Community-supported Agriculture (CSA) program. The concept of CSA programs, having begun only in the mid-1980s in the U.S., is relatively new to U.S. agriculture. CSAs originated in the 1960s in Japan, where a group of women concerned about the increase in food imports and the diminishing number of farms began to buy directly from local farms. The arrangement, called "teikei" in Japanese, translates to "putting the farmers' face on food."

When you buy food at the supermarket, it is estimated that your food has traveled between 1,500 and 2,500 miles from the farm to the market shelf, as much as 25 percent farther than in 1980. Almost every state in the U.S. buys 85–90 percent of its food from someplace else, according to a University of Massachusetts analysis. Enrolling in a CSA can help put you in better touch with where your food comes from and let you discover foods being grown seasonally in your state or community. CSAs can dramatically reduce the "food miles" of the items in your pantry and promote local and regional food production.

There are currently more than 1,000 CSA farms in the U.S. and Canada, with most located near urban centers in New England, the Mid-Atlantic states, and the Great Lakes region.[13] These innovative farming operations are taking off in America's big cities like New York, where an estimated 6,000 New Yorkers, including many in the poorer parts of the city, have joined together in buying clubs in just the last few years to get organic vegetables fresh from the farm throughout the growing season.[14] A growing number, are being established in other areas around the country, including on the West Coast.

A CSA works similar to buying stock in a company. To join a CSA, you buy a share of the harvest. As a shareholder, you receive a portion of the food produced each year from the farm. The amount you receive depends on the extent of the farm's bounty. In addition to owning part of the farm's produce, you also have the opportunity to visit the farm and work on it to better understand exactly how the food is grown. At some CSAs, you can even work off a portion of your share. Spending a day learning about where your food comes from, the hard work needed to grow the food, and the remarkable skill and knowledge of your local farmer can be a great learning experience for adults and children alike.

In most cases, CSAs extend over the entire growing season in your region. Members sign up and buy their share at the beginning of the growing season—usually in one lump sum, although sometimes installments are available. Most CSAs offer a diversity of vegetables, fruits, and herbs in season; some provide a full array of farm produce, including shares in eggs, meat, milk, baked goods, and even firewood. And every week you will pick up, or have delivered to a distribution point, a box full of fresh food produced at the farm the previous week. Weekly shares vary by size and types of produce, reflecting local growing seasons and conditions. Most shares are designed to meet the produce needs of a family of four for one week. But in many cases, what you get is far too much food for one family or household, and you'll find yourself either learning to can or preserve your surplus, or else sharing your weekly CSA bounty with friends or coworkers.

To tap into an increasing demand from consumers for fresh food alternatives, USDA's Sustainable Agriculture Network (SAN) has assembled a list of CSA farms nationwide. Available in print as well as on the World Wide Web, the list of more than 500 farms offers names and contact information for CSA operations in almost every state. To access the new CSA list, see www.sare.org/csa/index.htm, where you can search by state.

WHY IS COMMUNITY-SUPPORTED AGRICULTURE IMPORTANT?

- CSA's direct marketing gives farmers and growers the fairest return on their products.
- CSA keeps food dollars in the local community and contributes to the maintenance and establishment of regional food production.
- CSA encourages communication and cooperation among farmers.
- With a "guaranteed market" for their produce, farmers can invest their time in doing the best job they can rather than looking for buyers.
- CSA supports the biodiversity of a given area and the diversity of agriculture through the preservation of small farms producing a wide variety of crops.
- CSA creates opportunity for dialogue between farmers and consumers.
- CSA creates a sense of social responsibility and stewardship of local land.
- CSA puts "the farmers' face on food" and increases understanding of how, where, and by whom our food is grown.

Source: UMass Extension Agroecology Program.

ANOTHER GREAT way to find non-GE organic food is at farmers' markets. The U.S. has seen an explosion of farmers' markets in the last ten years. USDA's National Farmers Market Directory listed just 656 in 1994. Now, the USDA estimates there are close to 3,100 farmers' markets—involving over 20,000 farmers—around the country.

While the approximately $1 billion in farmers' market sales is a fraction of the $300 billion in U.S. agricultural sales, the small figure represents direct sales from farmers to consumers—with no corporate middleman.[15]

These markets can usually be found in urban areas—where farmers outside the city have come to a common location to sell their produce. For example, in New York City, Greenmarket now runs 28 different farmers' markets.

Farmers' markets give you an opportunity to actually meet the farmer growing your food. While you're there, you can ask him or her about the growing practices. Many farmers at farmers' markets are using organic methods and most are not using genetically engineered seeds—but you should always ask if the farmer is certified organic.

Farmers' markets are also a big part of the Women, Infants, and Children (WIC) Program. In 1992, WIC established its Farmers Market Program to provide fresh, nutritious, unprepared foods, such as fruit and vegetables, from farmers to people who are nutritionally at risk and to expand the awareness and use of farmers markets by consumers. The use of food stamps at farmers' markets nationwide is huge—estimated at $20.8 million in 2002, according to the USDA. During fiscal year 2002, over 2.1 million WIC participants received benefits for the Farmers' Markets Program.

Additionally, sales from farmers' markets to school meals programs are being promoted by USDA's Agricultural Marketing Service, Rural Development, and Food and Nutrition Service in California, Florida, Georgia, and North Carolina.

USDA makes it easy to find a listing of the farmers' markets in your state. Go to www.ams.usda.gov/farmersmarkets/index.htm and click on a picture of your state to bring up an alphabetical listing.

JOIN A BUYING CLUB

WHOLESALE BUYING clubs are yet another resource for organic and natural products and dry goods. Thousands of organic and natural food buying clubs have now sprung up across the country—both in rural and urban areas. The eight wholesale distributors listed below deliver food to buying clubs as well as supplying retail consumer co-ops and supply co-ops. Buying clubs are groups of people who join together and purchase foods and other grocery items in bulk at considerable savings. By buying in bulk or combining their order, buying clubs can often save you 10–50 percent off retail prices on organic and natural food products. This basically means that you can buy the highest quality organic food through your buying club at prices cheaper than conventional foods in your local supermarket. A buying club can be as small as one or two households within a city block or as large as one thousand households in a hundred mile radius. Many times, buying clubs are informal organizations made up of friends, family, coworkers, church groups, and other associations. You may also be able to join an existing buying club in your area. Contact one of the wholesalers below to find out whether there is a buying club in your area.

United Natural Foods—Blooming Prairie
  2340 Heinz Road
  Iowa City, IA 52240
  Fax: 319–337–4592
  Phone: 319–337–6448
  Web site: www.blooming-prairie.com/

United Natural Foods—Blooming Prairie
510 Kasota Avenue SE
Minneapolis,MN
Phone: 612–378–9774
Web site: www.blooming-prairie.com/

North Farm Cooperative
204 Regas Road
Madison, WI 53714
Fax: 608–241–0688
Phone:1–800–236–5880
Web site: www.northfarm-coop.com
Serves Indiana, Ohio, Minnesota, Wisconsin, Kentucky,
Missouri, Illinois, Michigan, North Dakota, Wyoming

United Northeast
Phone: 800–451–2525
Web site: www.unitednortheast.com

Frontier Natural Products Coop
2990 Wilderness Place Suite 200
Boulder, CO 80301
Fax: 303–449–8139
Phone: 303–449–8137
Web site: www.frontiercoop.com

Ozark Cooperative Warehouse
P.O. Box 1528
Fayetteville, AR 72702
Fax: 501–521–9100
Phone: 501–521–4920
Web site: www.ozarkcoop.com
Serves Alaska, Arkansas, Florida, Georgia, Kansas, Louisiana,
Michigan, Mississippi, Oklahoma, South Carolina, Tennessee,
and Texas

Tucson Cooperative Warehouse
  350 S. Toole Avenue
  Tucson, AZ 85701
  Fax: 520–792–3241
  Phone: 800–350–2667
  Web site: www.tcwfoodcoop.com
  Serves Arkansas, New Mexico, west Texas, southern California,
    southern Nevada, Utah, and Colorado.

ORDER ORGANIC AND NATURAL FOOD ON LINE

A GROWING trend in buying organic and natural food is through online services. Several national online supermarkets deliver a wide variety of vegetables, as well as meat and dairy products, to your home through the mail. Although buying from national locations like these has yet to become widespread, they offer an extensive selection of organic foods, and it is a great way to buy otherwise hard-to-find organic specialty foods and ingredients.

In addition, in several cities including Atlanta, Seattle, and Chicago, you can find delivery services for organic and natural foods. These services are able to provide fresh produce—mostly from local farmers—and often other food items as well, such as dairy and meat.

Here is a short list of places where you can buy organic produce online, as well as local delivery services:

MotherNature.Com
  Phone: 1–800–517–9020
  Web site: www.mothernature.com
  Offers dry goods such as vitamin, supplements, baby products,
    bath and beauty products, herbs, natural home supplies, cof-
    fee, tea, and cleaning products.

Sunshine Organic Foods
P.O. Box 258
Watsonville, CA 95077
Phone: 831–728–9218
Web site: www.sunshineorganic.com
Complete selection of natural and conventional groceries—
shop online for delivery in the San Diego metro area.

Pioneer Organics
102½ NW 36th
Seattle, WA 98107
Phone: 206–632–3424
Fax: 206–632–0609
Web site: www.pioneerorganics.com
Seattle area service—"The Puget Sound's premier organic pro-
duce home delivery service." Variety boxes delivered year-
round with 100-percent-certified organic produce. Weekly or
biweekly delivery available. Order online.

Urban Organic
230A 7th Street
Brooklyn, NY 11215
Phone: 718–499–4321
Fax: 718–499–3188
Web site: www.urbanorganic.net
Ships boxes of organic produce nationwide, except for Alaska
and Hawaii. In addition to fruit and vegetable boxes, also
offers organic groceries, fresh-baked bread, soy products,
herbs and spices, dairy products, desserts, and more. Free
shipping in most areas.

Planet Organics
915 Cole St #172
San Francisco, CA 94117
Phone: 1–800–956–5855 or 415–522–0526
Fax: 415–648–2597
Web site: www.planetorganics.com/
Home and office delivery of organic produce in San Francisco
Bay area.

Green Grocer
Washington, DC
Phone: 301–565–1680
Web site: www.washingtonsgreengrocer.com/
Delivers farm-fresh organic produce, including eggs and dairy.

GROW YOUR OWN!

WHEN YOU decide to grow your own produce, the rewards go well beyond great food. While you probably can't grow all your food, you'd be surprised how many vegetables—both in numbers and variety—you can grow in most climates in the U.S. Growing food in your backyard can be especially enjoyable because it helps strengthen and diversify your own backyard ecosystem.

Organic gardeners usually start off by building up healthy, rich soil fed constantly with organic matter—such as material from your compost pile—including kitchen scraps, leaves, and animal manure. Improved soil adds valuable nutrients, loosens clay-based soil, and improves drainage. Organic gardening also usually involves extensive mulching crop rotation, and often integrates herbs, flowers, and vegetables. Certain flowers like marigolds, pansies, and scented geraniums deter pests such as aphids, Japanese beetles, nematodes, snails, and slugs.

By not using toxic pesticides in your garden, you avoid killing bugs and beneficial insects like bees and ladybugs, ground beetles, lacewings, and spiders. There are several effective natural pest controls (such as milky spore for Japanese beetle grubs and Deer Off for deer). Many organic gardeners also employ homemade treatments such as soap spray for aphids, a mixture of yeast and sugar water for slugs, and hot-pepper spray for other pests. Or they may use "floating row cover," which is fabric, similar to cheesecloth, that covers plants and is porous to air, water, and sunlight, but not insects. An option of last resort is a bottle of Bt, (Bacillus thuringiensis), the non–genetically engineered variety, of course, in organic spray form.

For tips, suggestions, and information on growing in your backyard, find an issue of the bible of organic gardening—*Organic Gardening Magazine*. Or see Maria Rodale's *Organic Gardening*. Information can be found at: www.organicgardening.com.

The Rodale Institute also has a plethora of information on organic gardening, including numerous books and articles, and a reference center for questions. For information on their books, give them a call at: 800–832–6285, or check out their Web site: www.rodaleinstitute.org.

Another excellent resource for gardeners is GardenWeb, which hosts a number of forums, including one on organic gardening. These forums answer questions, acquire seeds, and offer gardening tips. The Web site is: www.gardenweb.com.

See Chapter 10 for additional gardening resources.

COMMUNITY GARDENS

IF YOU live in a city and don't have your own yard or land to garden, look for a community garden. An estimated 10,000 community gardens now grace U.S. cities nationwide. Community gardens have the added benefit of bringing your community closer together.

For more information about how to start and run a community garden, check in with the American Community Gardening Association (ACGA)—a national, nonprofit membership organization of professionals, volunteers, and supporters of community gardens in both urban and rural communities. The ACGA has a searchable database online to locate community gardens nationwide. The ACGA also hosts a listserve that helps answer common questions about community gardening.

American Community Garden Network
100 N 20th Street, 5th Floor
Philadelphia, PA 19103-1495
Phone: 215–988–8785
Fax: 215–988–8810
Web site: www.communitygarden.org/

Another group to check in with is the Urban Community Garden Web site. It contains links to locating resources and community gardening organizations in your community: www.mind-spring.com/~communitygardens/.

ORGANIC SEEDS

WHEN GROWING your own food, make sure to buy organic or natural seeds, particularly traditional heirloom seeds, also known as open-pollinated or standard seeds. High quality seeds help to ensure biodiversity and protect the vibrancy of your garden. Organic seeds are the only seeds guaranteed to be GE-free.

Open-pollinated seeds propagate themselves by pollinating themselves or other plants. Pollination is carried out by wind, insects, or other natural carrying agents. During open-pollination, pollen is constantly being exchanged among dozens, or hundreds, or even thousands of plants that vary slightly genetically. The mixing of genetic material maintains the vibrancy of particular strains of plants—their ability to fight off disease and adapt to ever changing environmental conditions.

Heirloom or open-pollinating seeds are available through a number of natural seed companies. There are several options for purchasing these seeds both through the mail and over the Internet. Ask your seed source whether their seeds are genetically engineered—particularly if you are growing potatoes or sweet corn. (See chapter 10 for a list of companies using organic seeds.)

One of the largest organic seed companies is Seeds of Change: 1–888–762–7333 (www.seedsofchange.com). They sell 100 percent non–genetically engineered seeds. Seed Savers Exchange is another seed source dedicated to helping backyard farmers retain the genetic diversity of seeds and grow non-GE vegetables and other plants. The exchange describes a number of seed varieties with traits developed outside of genetic engineering. See chapter 10 for additional seed companies that have organic or natural seeds.

Johnny's Selected Seeds in Maine (www.johnnyseeds.com) is one of eight companies in New England, and forty in the U.S. and Canada, to sign on to the Safe Seed Initiative, a project launched by heirloom seed grower Tom Stearns (High Mowing Organic Seeds, Wolcott, VT, 802–888–1800) with the assistance of Vermont-NOFA (Northeast Organic Farming Association) (www.nofavt.org) and the Boston-based Council for Responsible Genetics (www.gene-watch.org). See chapter 7 for a list of companies that have signed the pledge.

RESTAURANTS

A GROWING number of chefs nationwide are striving to buy and serve locally and organically produced foods. In fact, several hundred of the nation's top chefs advocate avoiding GE foods and ingredients and using organic ingredients whenever possible. Some of these top chefs include: Alice Waters (Chez Panisse Café and Restaurant, Café Fanny, Berkeley, CA), Nora Pouillon (Restaurant Noras, Washington, DC), Rick Bayless (Topolobampo and Frontera Grill, Chicago), Jesse Cool (Flea Street Cafe, Menlo

Park, CA), Stan Frankenthaler (Salamander Restaurant, Cambridge), Peter Hoffman (Savoy, New York), Lucia Watson (Lucias Restaurant and Wine Bar, Minneapolis), and Charlie Trotter (Charlie Trotters, Chicago).

Many of these top chefs leading this new wave of cooking are a part of the nationwide network called the Chefs Collaborative. The Chefs Collaborative (www.chefscollaborative.org) has over 1,500 chefs nationwide helping to promote sustainable cuisine by teaching children, supporting local farmers, educating one another, and inspiring the public to choose good, clean food.

The Chefs Collaborative works to improve recycling in kitchens, donating food to the hungry, buying locally, and buying organic food. Chefs Collaborative is now working closely with schools on an education program that teaches children where their food comes from and how it is prepared. The Adopt-a-School Program introduces kids to ways to eat healthy and protect their planet, and it incorporates the foods, culture, geography, and history of eight world regions (one of which is their own local region).

Chefs Collaborative has come out publicly in calling for the labeling of genetically engineered foods.[16]

Many of the nation's top chefs are going beyond simply trying to use organic ingredients, and are actively quizzing their suppliers on genetically engineered ingredients. Alice Waters of Chez Panisse has told her suppliers that her restaurant will be GE-free. At Seattle's Dahlia Lounge, chef Matt Costello has eliminated most genetically modified ingredients and is moving toward a total ban. In Philadelphia, the White Dog Cafe is also working toward a total ban. In April 2000, nearly 30 chefs in Philadelphia held a press conference denouncing GE technology and demanding labeling.

Among restaurateurs, Nora Pouillon has followed the emerging emphasis on organic food most thoroughly. Her Washington, D.C., restaurant, Restaurant Nora, is the only one in the country to be certified organic—95 percent of her ingredients are organic. Others in the industry are taking note: Pouillon won the "Award of Excellence" in the "Chef of the Year" category at the annual

International Association for Culinary Professionals 1997 Awards Ceremony.

These leading chefs are not alone in their search for organic food and ingredients. In Food & Wine magazine's 1997 Chef's Survey, 76 percent of chefs surveyed responded "Yes" to the question "Do you actively seek out organically grown ingredients?"

9

HOW YOU CAN SHOP
AND ACT WITH PURPOSE

GENETICALLY ENGINEERED food has slipped into our kitchens, lunchrooms, and restaurants quietly—without the knowledge of most consumers. It is unlikely this new technology will leave our shelves in the same quiet manner. It is up to us to let food companies, supermarkets, and the biotech industry know that we don't want these "novel" foods. It will take an informed and concerted consumer action—both at home and in the body politic—to pressure U.S. regulatory agencies to become more vigilant. And we need to demand that our elected representatives put forth a policy on genetically engineered foods that ensures the food supply is safe and that gives consumers all pertinent information about exactly what we are eating.

AS A food consumer, every dollar you spend on food not only has practical value helping to feed you and your family, but also delivers a political and economic message about what kind of agricultural system you support. In effect, you vote every time you buy food. Every dollar you spend on processed food, junk food, or genetically engineered food sends one message. But every dollar you spend on organic or natural food, locally grown food, or on food grown outside of the supermarket system (in farmers' markets, CSAs, co-ops, etc.) sends another message—that you want food to be safe, fresh, and environmentally friendly. As we've already discussed, the food industry is slowly starting to "get it" and is introducing a wide array of organic food products and standing against biopharm crops. But it is up to all of us to push the industry further by spending our consumer dollars responsibly.

Aside from trying to avoid purchasing genetically engineered foods, there are several other small but significant steps you can take at your grocery store. The most effective way to influence your local grocer or a particular food company is to write a letter or e-mail directly to its corporate headquarters. While letters or e-mails take time to write, they hold the greatest weight among companies. Companies are obligated to respond—and if you ask them specific questions, it is more difficult for them to respond with a form letter. Ask the companies whether they sell genetically engineered foods and how they identify which foods contain genetically engineered ingredients, and demand that they make more information available for consumers. You can also call them on the telephone on their toll-free "consumer comment" lines and request that they put their policies on genetically engineered foods in writing. A list of America's 25 major food companies and contact information is available in chapter 6 and the Organic Consumer Association has posted a list of the phone numbers of the "Frankenfoods 15," leading American food companies that have refused to guarantee that their foods are GE-free, on the Internet at www.organicconsumers.org/cando.htm

GET YOUR SCHOOL TO GO GE-FREE

WHILE COMMON sense tells us that the food we feed our children should be the safest and most nutritious available, a trip to the school lunchroom often tells a different story. In fact, most schools offer more junk food than ever—soft drinks, candy bars, and a wide variety of processed, packaged food. This growing menu of generally unhealthy food is increasing at shocking rates nationwide.

It is important to remember that your tax dollars support your schools. Local school boards offer an opportunity to affect what the children of your community are fed each day for lunch. In every part of the country, there are opportunities to limit exposures to genetically engineered food by following the recommendations outlined in this book.

Changes are beginning to take place. The school district in Berkeley, California, has already acted to dramatically change its school lunch program. After concerned parents visited school officials regarding the district's school lunch program, Berkeley schools developed a lunch program that bans the use of genetically engineered foods, irradiated foods, and dairy products from cows injected with the recombinant Bovine Growth Hormone (rBGH). Other goals of the district's plan include establishing a child nutrition advisory committee and eliminating food additives and high-fat, high-sugar snacks and entrees.

In addition, Berkeley has offered organic food for lunch. Administrators hope to defray some of the added expense of purchasing organic foods by growing sixteen percent of the produce on the campuses themselves. Eleven of Berkeley's 16 schools already have gardens.

In the last few years, this movement has taken off. Ross School and Bridgehampton School on Long Island have a school lunch program with organic and locally grown foods. Kemberton Waldorf School in Pennsylvania serves organic and vegetarian lunches. Organic milk is dispensed in milk machines in upstate New York schools. Three Sante Fe, New Mexico, schools get a salad bar from local produce. The New North Florida Co-op of farmers sells local produce to 13 schools in Florida, Georgia, and Alabama. Decorah, Iowa, buys locally grown produce for salad bars and a la carte items. Locally grown watermelons, sweet potatoes, and broccoli are served to children in Clark County, Kentucky. The National Farm to School Program, funded through the USDA, now has programs in California, Pennsylvania, New York, and New Jersey. For more information, go to: www.farmtoschool.org

LEGISLATING TO PROTECT CONSUMERS

MOST U.S. legislators know very little about genetically engineered foods and their potential threats to human health and the environment. It is absolutely critical that we let our legislators know of our concerns about the environmental and human health threats of genetically engineered foods and the lack of available pertinent information for consumers about these foods.

The biotech and food industry have spent large amounts of money in campaign contributions to influence legislators on this issue. In the 2002 election cycle, Monsanto and its parent company Pharmacia gave over $1.4 million in political contributions, according to the Center for Public Integrity. Also in 2002, Syngenta gave over $380,000 in contributions, Dow Chemical over $450,000, and the Biotechnology Industry Organization (BIO) over $130,000. Contacting your U.S. congressperson or state representatives is not difficult. In fact, most legislators want to hear from their constituents. Letter writing is the best way to communicate your concerns. Each letter sent to a legislator is counted and tracked. Of course, phone calls and e-mails are also effective ways to communicate with your legislator. If you have time, it is always worthwhile to set up a meeting with your representative or his or her staff to discuss your concerns.

As we discussed in chapter 5, a number of innovative legislative measures are being introduced to address genetically engineered foods, at the national, state, and local levels. Find out where your state and federal legislators stand on these issues and urge them to take action if they haven't already done so.

OUR REGULATORY SYSTEM

THE FOOD and Drug Administration (what we eat), the Environmental Protection Agency (the environment), and the U.S. Department of Agriculture (what we grow) regulate genetically engineered foods. (For more details, see chapter 5.) As federal entities, they operate under the president and the cabinet secretaries he appoints. It is important that consumers let those at regulatory agencies and the president know that GE crops are not adequately regulated and that immediate steps need to be taken to ensure the safety of human health and the environment.

All three regulatory agencies routinely engage in what is called the "rule-making" process, and frequently ask for public input on a number of agency policies. The Web sites of all three agencies (www.fda.gov, www.epa.gov, www.usda.gov) provide timely information and opportunities for public comment. Keep an eye out for opportunities to submit your own comments to these agencies regarding their policies on genetically engineered foods and other food and agriculture issues. Public comments can have a big impact at agencies. For instance, when the USDA proposed national organic rules that were riddled with harmful loopholes, nearly 300,000 citizens submitted comments. The agency scrapped the first proposed rules and rewrote them—paying special attention to citizens' comments.

ORGANIZATIONS AND CAMPAIGNS

IF YOU'RE ready to become more active on the issue of genetic engineering, there are a number of organizations and campaigns that could use your help. A great way to get plugged in is to join one of the following groups and their campaigns:

- Friends of the Earth—Friends of the Earth's Safer Food, Safer Farms campaign is targeting U.S. federal agencies to better regulate GE foods and crops. FOE has called for a moratorium on further releases into the environment of all GE crops. FOE is organizing demonstrations outside major supermarket chains, calling on the stores to remove all GE ingredients from their own brand labels, and has particularly targeted Kraft. FOE is also working with shareholders to hold food and biotech corporations accountable. For more information on FOE's Safer Food, Safer Farms campaign, visit their Web site at: www.foe.org.
- Greenpeace USA—Greenpeace has been a leading opponent worldwide to genetically engineered foods. In the U.S., Greenpeace has sued the EPA regarding the environmental impacts of genetically engineered crops, successfully convinced Gerber baby foods to go GE-free, and targeted a number of other U.S. food companies through protests and other actions. Visit their Web site at: www.greenpeaceusa.org/ge.
- Organic Consumers Association—The OCA is a nationwide network of 500,000 organic consumers, challenging GMOs and industrial farming and promoting organic agriculture and fair trade. OCA organizes within food co-ops and natural food stores and among consumers of organic food in all 50 states. OCA helps organize consumers to submit comments to federal agencies, safeguard organic standards, and directly target food companies that use genetically engineered ingredients. OCA is currently targeting what it calls the "Frankenfoods 15"—food companies that are using GE technology. For more information, call 218–226–4164, or go to: www.organicconsumers.org.
- Foundation on Economic Trends—Run by long-time biotech opponent Jeremy Rifkin this organization recently organized

a massive lawsuit against Monsanto and other biotech companies, charging that they were violating U.S. antitrust laws. This vital lawsuit directly challenges the biotech industry and their attempt to control all aspects of agriculture. For more information, visit www.foet.org.

- Center for Food Safety—The Center is a nonprofit legal firm in Washington, D.C., has filed two ground-breaking lawsuits against U.S. regulatory agencies. The first challenges the FDA's policy on genetically engineered foods, demanding that the agency require safety testing and labeling of these foods. The second challenges the EPA's regulation of genetically engineered Bt crops, calling for the agency to conduct more thorough analysis of risks before the products enter the market. For more information go to: www.centerforfoodsafety.org. (For an additional listing of organizations, Web sites, and other information resources, see chapter 10.)

- The Genetic Engineering Action Network—is a diverse network of grassroots activists, national and community nongovernmental organizations (NGOs), farmer and farm advocacy groups, academics, and scientists who have come together to work on the myriad of issues surrounding biotechnology. On the Web at: www.geaction.org.

10

WHERE TO FIND OUT MORE

OTHER BOOKS ON GENETIC ENGINEERING

Fox, Michael, *Eating with Conscience: The Bioethics of Food* (NewSage Press, 1997).

Hart, Kathleen. *Eating in the Dark, America's Experiment with Genetically Engineered Food* (Pantheon Books, 2002).

Ho, Mae-Wan, *Genetic Engineering: Dream or Nightmare* (Gateway Books, 1998).

Jack, Alex, *Imagine a World Without Monarch Butterflies* (One Peaceful World Press, 1999).

Kimbrell, Andrew, *The Human Body Shop: The Engineering and Marketing of Life* (HarperCollins, 1993).

Kneen, Brewster, *Farmageddon: Food and the Culture of Biotechnology,* (New Society Publishers, 1999).

Lambrecht, Bill. *Dinner at the New Gene Café* (Thomas Dunne Books, 2001).

Lappe, Mark and Britt Baily, *Against the Grain* (Common Courage Press, 1998).

Nottingham, S., *Eat Your Genes: How Genetically Modified Food Is Entering Our Diet* (Zed Books, 1998).

Rifkin, Jeremy, *The Biotech Century* (Tarcher/Putnam, 1998).

Shiva, Vandana, *Biopiracy: The Plunder of Nature and Knowledge* (South End Press, 1997).

Smith, Jeffrey. *Seeds of Deception* (Yes! Books, 2003).

Teitel, Martin and Kimberly A. Wilson, *Genetically Engineered Food: Changing the Nature of Nature* (Park Street Press, 1999).

Ticciati, Laura and Robin Ticcati, *Genetically Engineered Foods: Are They Safe? You Decide* (Keats, 1998).

Turney, Jon, *Frankenstein's Footsteps: Science, Genetics and Popular Culture* (Yale University Press, 1998).

ORGANIZATIONS AND WEB SITES

Genetically Engineered Foods

National
Ag Biotech Info-Net
Web site: www.biotech-info.net/

Alliance for Bio-Integrity
406 W Depot Avenue
Fairfield, IA 52556
Phone: 515–472–5554
Web site: www.bio-integrity.org

Campaign to Label Genetically Engineered Foods
P.O. Box 55699
Seattle, WA 98155
Phone: 425–771–4049
Web site: www.thecampaign.org

Center for Ethics and Toxics
39141 S Highway 1
P.O. Box 673
Gualala, CA 95445
Phone: 707–884–1700
Web site: www.cetos.org

Center for Food Safety
66 Pensylvania Ave SE Suite#302
Washington, DC 20003
Phone: 202–547–9359
Web site: www.centerforfoodsafety.org

Citizens for Health
   Web site: www.citizens.org

Consumers Union
   101 Truman Avenue
   Yonkers, NY 10703
   Phone: 914–378–2452
   Web site: www.consumersunion.org/i/Food_Safety/

Council for Responsible Genetics
   5 Upland Road, Suite 3
   Cambridge, MA 02140
   Phone: 617–868–0870
   Web site: www.gene-watch.org

Cropchoice
   P.O. Box 33811
   Washington, D.C. 20033
   Phone: 202–797–7554
   Web site: www.cropchoice.com

The Edmonds Institute
   20319 92nd Avenue West
   Edmonds, WA 98020
   Phone: 425–775–5383
   Web site: www.edmonds-institute.org

Environmental Defense
   257 Park Avenue South
   New York, NY 10010
   Phone: 800–684–3322
   Web site: www.environmentaldefense.org

Foundation on Economic Trends
   1660 L Street NW, Suite 216
   Washington DC 20036
   Phone: 202–466–2823
   Web site: www.foet.org/

Friends of the Earth
   1717 Massachusetts Avenue, NW, 600
   Washington, DC 20036–2002
   Phone: 202–783–7400, 877–843–8687
   Web site: www.foe.org

Genetic Engineering Action Network (GEAN)
11 Ward St. Suite 200
Somerville, MA 02143
Phone: 617–661–6626
Web site: www.geaction.org

Genetically Engineered Food Alert
Web site: gefoodalert.org/pages/home.cfm

Greenpeace USA
564 Mission Street
P.O. Box 416
San Francisco, CA 94105
Phone: 800–326–0959
Web site: www.greenpeaceusa.org/ge/

Institute for Agriculture and Trade Policy
2105 1st Avenue South
Minneapolis, MN 55404
Phone: 612–870–0453
Web site: www.iatp.org

Mothers for Natural Law
P.O. Box 1900
Fairfield, IA 52556
515–472–2040
Web site: www.safe-food.org

Non-GMO Source
Web site: www.non-gmosource.com

Organic Consumers Association
6101 Cliff Estate Road
Little Marais, MN 55614
Phone: 218–226–4164
Web site: www.organicconsumers.org/

True Fo'od Network
Web site: www.truefoodnow.org

Union of Concerned Scientists
2 Brattle Square
Cambridge, MA 02238–9105
Phone: 617–547–5552
Web site: www.ucsusa.org

U.S. Public Interest Research Group (PIRG)
218 D Street, SE
Washington, D.C. 20003
Phone: 202–546–9707
Web site: www.uspirg.org

Regional/Local
Colorado Genetic Engineering Action Network
1140 US Hwy 287
Suite 400-125
Broomfield, CO 80020
303–215–3384
Web site: www.foodlabeling.org/index.asp

Florida Alliance for Safe Foods
P.O. Box 21511
Sarasota, FL 34276–4511
Phone: 941–362–3869
Web site: protectorganic.org/sasf/index.htm

North Carolina Citizens for Safe Food
Web site: www.purefoodpartners.org/

Northeast Resistance Against Genetic Engineering
Vermont Clearinghouse
c/o Institute for Social Ecology
1118 Maple Hill Road
Plainfield, VT 05667
Phone: 802–454–9957
Web site: www.nerage.org/

NW RAGE
P.O. Box 15289
Portland, OR 97293
Phone: 503–236–5772, ext. 2
Web site: www.nwrage.org/nwrage.html

Gateway Greens
P.O. Box 8094
St. Louis, MO 63156
Phone: 314–771–8576
Web site: www.greens.org/s-r/gga/

Rural Vermont
15 Barre Street
Montpelier, VT 05602
Phone: 802–223–7222
Web site: www.greenfornewengland.org/

ETC Group—Action Group on Erosion, Technology and Concentration
Web site: www.etcgroup.org

Institute of Science in Society (ISIS)
Web site: www.i-sis.org.uk/

Physicians and Scientists for Responsible Application of Science and Technology (PSRAST)
Web site: www.pcrm.org

Third World Network
Web site: www.twnside.org.sg

Pesticides

Community Alliance with Family Farmers CA
P.O. Box 363
Davis, CA 95617
Phone: 530–756–8518
Web site: www.caff.org

International Federation of Organic Agriculture Movements (IFOAM)
Web site: www.ifoam.org

National Campaign for Sustainable Agriculture
P.O. Box 396
Pine Bush, NY 12566
Phone: 845–361–5201
Web site: www.sustainableagriculture.net/

National Coalition Against the Misuse of Pesticides
701 E Street, SE, Suite 200
Washington, DC 20003
Phone: 202–543–5450
Web site: www.beyondpesticides.org

Organic Alliance
400 Selby Avenue, Suite T
St. Paul, MN 55102
Phone: 651–265–3678
Web site: www.organic.org

Organic Consumers Association
6101 Cliff Estate Road
Little Marais, MN 55614

Phone: 218–226–4164
Web site: www.organicconsumers.org

Organic Farm Research Foundation
P.O. Box 440
Santa Cruz, CA 95061
Phone: 831–426–6606
Web site: www.ofrf.org

Organic Materials Review Institute
Box 11558
Eugene, OR 97440–3758
Phone: 541–343–7600
Web site: www.omri.org

Organic Trade Association
74 Fairview Street
P.O. Box 547
Greenfield, MA 01302
Phone: 413–774–7511
Web site: www.ota.com

Pesticide Action Network of North America
49 Powell St, Suite 500
San Francisco, CA 94102
Phone: 415–981–1771
Web site: www.panna.org

Rodale Institute
611 Siegfriedale Road
Kutztown, PA 19530
Phone: 610–683–1400 (experimental farm), 800-832-6285 (bookstore)
Web site: www.rodaleinstitute.org

Rural Advancement Foundation International (USA)
P.O. Box 640
Pittsboro, NC 27312
Phone: 919–542–1396
Web site: http://www.rafiusa.org/

USDA National Organic Program
Web site: www.ams.usda.gov/nop

Community-supported Agriculture Programs

CSAs by state
Web site: www.umass.edu/umext/csa

Farmers' Market Online
Web site: www.farmersmarketonline.com/communit.htm

Organic Consumers Association
Web site: www.organicconsumers.org/csa.htm

Sustainable Agriculture Network
Web site: www.sare.org/csa/index.htm

USDA Alternative Farming Systems Information Center
Web site: www.nal.usda.gov/afsic/csa/

Farmers' Markets

California Federation of Certified Farmers' Markets
Web site: www.cafarmersmarkets.com/

Colorado Farmers' Markets
Web site: www.ag.state.co.us/mkt/farmfresh/2003/farmersmarkets.html

Farmers' Markets
Web site: www.farmersmarketonline.com/index.html

Federation of Massachusetts Farmers' Markets
Web site: www.massfarmersmarkets.org/

Iowa Farmers' Market Directory
Web site: www.agriculture.state.ia.us/farmermarket.asp

Jersey Fresh
Web site: www.state.nj.us/jerseyfresh/searches/urban.htm

Local Harvest
Web site: www.localharvest.org

Maine Federation of Farmers' Markets
Web site: home.gwi.net/~troberts/mffm/

Missouri Alternatives Center
Web site: http://agebb.missouri.edu/mac/

National Directory of Fruit Stands and Farmers' Markets
Web site:www.fruitstands.com/

New Hampshire Farmers' Market Association
Web site: http://nhfma.bizland.com/

New Mexico Farmers' Marketing Association
Web site: www.farmersmarketsnm.org

New York Farmers' Markets
Web site: www.nyfarmersmarket.com/

New York's Just Food
Web site: www.justfood.org

North Carolina Farmers' Markets
Web site:www.ncagr.com/markets/facilit/farmark/

Oregon Farmers' Market Association
Web site: www.oregonfarmersmarkets.org/

Resources for Farmers' Markets
Web site: www.nemw.org/farmersmarkets/

The Small Farm Program—USDA Cooperative State, Research, Education, and
Extension Service
Web site: www.reeusda.gov/smallfarm

Sustainable Agriculture Network
Web site: www.sare.org

Tennessee Farmers' Markets
Web site: www.picktnproducts.org/produce/farmers.html

Texas Farmers' Markets
Web site: www.agr.state.tx.us/picktexas/farm_market/farmers_market2.htm

Urban Agriculture Notes/City Farmer—Canada's Office of Urban Agriculture
Web site: www.cityfarmer.org

USDA's Farmers' Market Source
Web site: www.ams.usda.gov/farmersmarkets/

Vermont Farmers' Markets
Web site: www.vermontagriculture.com/farmmkt.htm

Washington State Farmers' Market Association
Web site: www.wafarmersmarkets.com/

Wisconsin Farmers' Markets
Web site: www.wisconline.com/attractions/farmmarkets.html

Community Gardening

American Community Garden Network
100 N 20th Street, 5th Floor
Philadelphia, PA 19103–1495
Phone: 215–988–8785
Fax: 215–988–8810
Web site: www.communitygarden.org/index.html

Co-ops

Co-op America
1612 K Street, NW, Suite 600
Washington, DC 20006
Web site: www.coopamerica.org

Co-op Network
P.O. Box 57
Randolph, VT 05060
Phone: 802–234–9293

Cooperative Development Institute
277 Federal Street
Greenfield, MA 01301
Phone: 413–774–7599
E-mail: info@cooplife.com
Web site: www.cooplife.com/

Cooperative Development Services
30 West Mifflin Street, Suite 401
Madison, WI 53703
Phone: 608–258–4396
E-mail: CDS@co-opdevelopmentservices.com
Web site: www.cdsus.coop/

Organic Consumers Association Food Co-op Directory
Web site: www.organicconsumers.org/storesearch.htm

Organic and Natural Seed Companies

Abundant Life Seed Foundation
P.O. Box 772
930 Lawrence Street
Port Townsend, WA 98368
Phone: 206–385–5660

E-mail: matthew@seedalliance.org
Web site: www.abundantlifeseed.org/
Rare grains, herbs, compost crops, and European heirlooms. Affiliated with
Ecology Action.

Burpee Heirloom Seed Catalog
W. Atlee Burpee Co.
300 Park Avenue
Warminister, PA 18991–0008
Phone: 800–999–8552
Web site: www.burpee.com
Untreated seed upon request (except corn).

Butterbrooke Farm
78 Barry Road
Oxford, CT 06483
Phone: 203–888–2000
Non-hybrid hardy vegetable strains raised by cooperating farmers. SASE for
price list.

Comstock Ferre
263 Main Street
Wethersfield, CT 06109
Phone: 860–571–6590
E-mail: canstock@tiac.net
Web site: www.comstockferre.com/

The Cook's Garden
P.O. Box 535
Londonderry, VT 05148
Phone: 800–457–9713
E-mail: orders@cooksgarden.com
Web site: www.cooksgarden.com

Dacha Barinka
46232 Strathcona Road
Chilliwack, BC V2P 3T2
Phone: 604–792–0957

Down on the Farm Seeds
P.O. Box 184
Hiram, OH 44234
Seedlist $1.00. Untreated heirloom/open-pollinated seed. By mail only.

Ed Hume Seeds, Inc.
P.O. Box 1450

Kent, WA 98035
Phone: 253–859–1110
E-mail: humeseeds@aol.com
Web site: www.humeseeds.com

Elixir Farm Botanicals
General Delivery
Brixey, MO 65618
Contact: Lavinia McKinney
Phone: 417–261–2393
E-mail: efb@aristotle.net
Web site: www.elixirfarm.com
Biodynamically certified organic seed of native and Chinese medicinal herbs.

Farmers Market Online
Web site: www.FarmersMarketOnline.com/index.html

FEDCO Seeds
P.O. Box 520
Waterville, ME 04903
Phone: 207–873–7333
Web site: www.fedcoseeds.com/
Seed cooperative.

Fox Hollow Seed Co.
P.O. Box 148
McGrann, PA 16236
Phone: 724–548–7333
Web site: www.foxhollowseed.com/

Fruited Plain Seeds
P.O. Box 56
Craigville, IN 46731
Phone: 219–565–3212
E-mail: smz@adamswells.com
Mostly cover crops. Also cleaning of food-grade seed for the organic industry.

Garden City Seeds
778 Hwy 93 N
Hamilton, MT 59840
Phone: 406–961–4837
E-mail: potatoes@irish-eyes.com
Web site: www.irish-eyes.com/
Trials and tests all Garden City vegetable varieties before offering for flavor, quick maturity, and vigor in the Far North. All seed is untreated, some organic.

Harris Seeds
   60 Saginaw Drive
   Rochester, NY 14692-2960
   Phone: 800–514–4441
   Web site: www.harrisseeds.com
   Offers some varieties untreated.

Heirloom Seeds
   P.O. Box 245
   West Elizabeth, PA 15088-0245
   Phone: 412–384–0852
   E-mail: mail@heirloomseeds.com
   Web site: www.heirloomseeds.com

Horizon Herbs
   P.O. Box 69
   Williams, OR 97544
   Phone: 541–846–6704
   Fax: 541–846–6233
   E-mail: herbseed@chatlink.com
   Web site: http://www.horizonherbs.com/

J. L. Hudson, Seedsman
   P.O. Box 1058
   Redwood City, CA 94064
   Web site: www.jlhudsonseeds.net/

Johnny's Selected Seeds
   184 Foss Hill Road
   P.O. Box 2580
   Albion, ME 04910
   Phone: 207–437–9294
   E-mail: johnnys@johnnyseeds.com
   Web site: www.johnnyseeds.com
   Treated (T) or Untreated (U) indicated. Medicinal herb section.

The KUSA Society
   P.O. Box 761
   Ojai, CA 93024

Heirloom Seed Project
   Landis Valley Museum
   2451 Kissel Hill Road
   Lancaster, PA 17601
   Phone: 717–569–0401
   Web site: www.landisvalleymuseum.org
   Single packets of heirloom varieties of the Pennsylvania Dutch.
   Untreated seed upon request.

Mighty Seed™
    Seed International, Inc.
    3208 Sue Circle
    Rio Rancho, NM 87124
    Phone: 505–892–7373 (request catalog)
    E-mail: jckf777@aol.com
    Garden seeds for sprouting, grains for human and animal consumption,
        kosher seeds, grains and bean varieties, and untreated and certified.

Moose Tubers
    P.O. Box 510
    Waterville, ME 04903
    Contact: Allison Lacourse
    Web site: www.fedcoseeds.com/moose.htm
    Division of FEDCO—see p. 219

Native Seeds/SEARCH
    526 N. 4th Avenue
    Tucson, AZ 85705–8450
    Phone: 520–622–5561 (no phone orders)
    Fax: 520–622–5591 (fax orders welcome)
    E-mail: info@nativeseeds.org
    Web site: www.nativeseeds.org/v2/default.php
    Native and traditional seeds of the Southwest. Nonprofit organization.
        Newsletter and publications.

The Natural Gardening Co.
    P.O. Box 750776
    Petaluma, CA 94975–0776
    Phone: 707–766–9303
    E-mail: info@naturalgardening.com
    Web site: www.naturalgardening.com
    Organically grown tomato seedlings and seeds of heirloom varieties.

Organic Consumers Association
    Web site: www.organicconsumers.org/seeds.htm

Peace Seeds
    P.O. Box 190
    Gila, NM 88038
    Web site: peaceseeds.elysiumgates.com/
    Jointly publishes Deep Diversity Catalog with Seeds of Change.

Pinetree Garden Seeds
    P.O. Box 300
    New Gloucester, ME 04260
    Phone: 207–926–3400

E-mail: superseeds@worldnet.att.net
Web site: www.superseeds.com

Plants of the Southwest
3095 Agua Fria Road
Santa Fe, NM 87507
Phone: 800–788–7333
E-mail: contact@pots.com
Web site: www.plantsofthesouthwest.com
Web site features 130 native wildflowers. Also herbs, vegetables.

Redwood City Seed Co.
P.O. Box 361
Redwood City, CA 94064
Phone: 650–325–7333
Web site: www.batnet.com/rwc-seed/index.html
Native seeds, open-pollinated vegetables. Pamphlets.

Ronniger's Seed Potatoes
P.O. Box 307
Ellensburg, WA 98926
Phone: 800-846-6178
E-mail: 103374.167@compuserve.com
Web site: http://ronnigers.com/
Large selection of organically grown seed potatoes.

Seed Dreams
P.O. Box 1476
Santa Cruz, CA 95061–1476
E-mail: sr012@csufresno.edu
Old-time heirloom vegetable and grain seeds, open-pollinated and organic.
    Will donate seeds to any children's gardening project.

Seed Savers Exchange
3076 North Winn Road
Decorah, IA 52101
Phone: 319–382–5990
Web site: www.seedsavers.org
All packets heirloom seed, $2.50/pkt.

Seeds of Change
P.O. Box 15700
Santa Fe, NM 87592
Phone: 888–762–7333
Web site: www.seedsofchange.com

Seeds of Diversity Canada
P.O. Box 36 Stn Q
Toronto, Ontario, M4T 2L7
Phone: 905–623–0353
E-mail: mail@seeds.ca
Web site: www.seeds.ca

Seeds West Garden Seeds
317 14th Street NW
Albuquerque, NM 87104
Phone: 505–843–9713
E-mail: seeds@nmia.com
Web site: www.seedswestgardenseeds.com
Heirloom garden seed for the Southwest. New owners 1998.

Southern Exposure Seed Exchange
P.O. Box 460
Mineral, VA 23117
Phone: 540–894–9480
E-mail: gardens@southernexposure.com
Web site: www.southernexposure.com
Catalog $2.00. Heirloom/open-pollinated seeds, alliums, fruit trees.

Stokes Seeds
P.O. Box 548
Buffalo, NY 14240–0548
Phone: 716–695–6980
E-mail: stokes@stokeseeds.com
Web site: www.stokeseeds.com
U.S. office of Canadian company; large selection, bulk (catalog not online).

Territorial Seed Company
P.O. Box 157
Cottage Grove, OR 97424–0061
Phone: 888–657–3131
E-mail: tetrl@srvl.vsite.com
Web site: www.territorial-seed.com

Thomas Jefferson Center for Historic Plants, Monticello
P.O. Box 318
Charlottesville, VA 22902
Web site: www.monticello.org/chp/

Thompson & Morgan
P.O. Box 1308
Jackson, NJ 08527–0308
Phone: 800–274–7333
E-mail: tminc@thompson-morgan.com
Web site: www.thompson-morgan.com
Large selection ornamental, vegetables.

Tomato Growers Supply Co.
P.O. Box 2237
Fort Myers, FL 33902
Phone: 941–768–1119 (customer service),
888–478–7333 (orders)
Fax: 888–768–3476
Web site: www.tomatogrowers.com
Heirloom tomatoes; most varieties untreated.

The Tomato Seed Co., Inc.
P.O. Box 323
Metuchen, NJ 08840
Phone: 201–548–9036
Heirloom tomatoes.

Turtle Enterprises
Route 1, Box 71
Dalton, WI 53926
SASE for catalog of sweet sorghum varieties.

White Flower Farm
P.O. Box 50, Route 63
Litchfield, Connecticut 06759
Phone: 800–503–9624
Web site: www.whiteflowerfarm.com/index.html
Mail-order source for plants, bulbs, and gardening supplies.

William Dam Seeds
P.O. Box 8400
279 Hwy 8 (West Flamboro)
Dundas, Ontario L9H 6M1
Phone: 905–628–6641
E-mail: willdam@damseeds.com
Web site: www.damseeds.com/
European, Oriental vegetables and houseplant seeds.

Organic Garden Fertilizer Sources

Garden Supplies

Bountiful Gardens
18001 Shafer Ranch Road
Willits, CA 95490–9626
Phone: 707–459–6410
E-mail: bountiful@zapcom.net
Web site: www.bountifulgardens.org
Catalogue sales, specializing in seed. Focus on biointensive farming and gardening. Good source for small quantities of hard-to-find covercrop seed.

Gardens Alive
5100 Schenley Place
Lawrenceburg, IN 47025
Phone: 812–537–8651 (customer service)
Web site: www.gardens-alive.com
Offers high-quality lawn and garden products that work with nature.

Harmony Farm Supply & Nursery
3244 Gravenstein Hwy N.
Sebastopol, CA 95472
Phone: 707–823–9125
E-mail: info@harmonyfarm.com
Web site: www.harmonyfarm.com
Primarily mail-order catalogue sales. Great diversity of offerings. Current catalogue: $2.00.

The Invisible Gardener
P.O. Box 4311
Malibu, CA 90265
Phone: 310–457–4438
Web site: www.invisiblegardener.com
For natural pest control and more.

Nitron Industries
P.O. Box 1447
Fayetteville, AR 72702
Phone: 800–835–0123
Web site: www.nitron.com
The premier source for organic fertilizers, soil amendments, non-hybrid seeds, and insect controls for lawns, gardens, and flower beds.

Organic Growers Supply
  P.O. Box 520
  Waterville, ME 04903
  Phone: 207–873–7333
  Web site: www.fedcoseeds.com/ogs.htm
  Primarily mail-order catalogue sales.

Peaceful Valley
  P.O. Box 2209
  Grass Valley, CA 95945
  Phone: 530–272–4769
  E-mail: contact@groworganic.com
  Web site: www.groworganic.com
  Primarily mail-order catalogue sales. Great diversity of offerings.
     Consulting service.

Planet Natural
  1612 Gold Avenue
  P.O. Box 3146
  Bozeman, MT 59772
  Phone: 406–587–5891 (information), 800–289–6656 (orders)
  E-mail: ecostore@mcn.net
  Web site: www.planetnatural.com
  Catalogue sales, specializing in natural pest controls.

Organic/Natural Meat

Coleman Natural Products Inc.
  5140 Race Court
  Denver, CO 80216
  Phone: 303–297–9393
  E-mail: coleman@colemannatural.com
  Web site: www.colemanmeats.com
  Available in many national grocery stores and coops. Find retail location
     closest to you on their Web site.

Laura's Lean Beef
  2285 Executive Drive, Suite 200
  Lexington, KY 40505
  Phone: 606–299–7707, 800–487–5326
  E-mail: llb@laurasleanbeef.com
  Web site: www.laurasleanbeef.com

Organic Valley Family of Farms—CROPP Cooperative
507 W. Main Street
La Farge, WI 54639
Phone: 888–444–6455
E-mail: organic@organicvalley.com
Web site: www.organicvalley.com

Miscellaneous

Seven Bridges Cooperative
419 May Avenue
Santa Cruz, CA 95060
800–769–4409
E-mail: 7bridges@breworganic.com
Web site: www.breworganic.com
Organic beer-brewing ingredients and supplies.

Organic Meat and Poultry

Eat Well Guide
Web site: www.eatwellguide.org

Organic Consumers Association
Web site: www.organicconsumers.org/organicfood.htm

Government

U.S. Department of Agriculture
Web site: www.aphis.usda.gov/brs/index.html

U.S. Environmental Protection Agency
Web site: www.epa.gov/scipoly/oscpbiotech.htm

U.S. Food and Drug Administration
Web site: www.cfsan.fda.gov/~lrd/biotechm.html

U.S. House of Representatives
Web site: www.house.gov

U.S. Senate
Web site: www.senate.gov

ENDNOTES

INTRODUCTION

1. For information on these polls see www.organicconsumers.org/gefood/polls051602.cfm and www.organicconsumers.org/ge/071703_ge.ctm
2. Marian Burros, "Biotechnology's Bounty," *New York Times* (May 21, 1997) and Marian Burros, "Eating Well: Genes are Changed, but Not the Label," *New York Times* (September 8, 1999).
3. Mike Hendricks, "Labels Not Required to Reveal All," *Kansas City Star* (March 7, 1994).

CHAPTER 1

1. Bill Hord, "Farmers Warned of Uncertainties With Crops Genetics," *Omaha World-Herald* (March 4, 2000).
2. Michael Hansen, "Genetic Engineering Is Not An Extension of Conventional Plant Breeding," Consumer Policy Institute (January 27, 2000). Submitted to the Food and Drug Administration.
3. Andrew Kimbrell, *The Human Body Shop: The Engineering and Making of Life,* (HarperCollins, 1993) p. 176.

4. J. Bergelson, C.B. Purrington, and G. Wichmann. 1998. "Promiscuity in transgenic plants." *Nature,* 395: 25.

5. T Inose, and K. Murata. 1995. "Enhanced Accumulation of Toxic Compound in Yeast Cells Having High Glycolytic Activity: A Case Study on the Safety of Genetically Engineered Yeast." *International Journal of Food Science and Technology,* 30: 141–146.

6. Michael Hansen, "Genetic Engineering Is Not An Extension of Conventional Plant Breeding," Consumer Policy Institute (January 27, 2000). Submitted to the Food and Drug Administration.

7. P. Meyer, F. Linn, I. Heidmann, H. Meyer, I. Niedenhof, and H. Saedler. 1992. "Endongenous and Environmental Factors Influence 35 S Promoter Methylation of a Maize A1 Gene Construct in Transgenic Petunia and Its Colour Phenotype." *Molecular Genes and Genetics,* 231: 345–352.

8. www.biotech-info.net/technicalpaper6.html

9. Ag Bio Tech InfoNet at www.biotech-info.net/RR_yield_drag_98.pdf

10. Charles Benbrook, "When Does It Pay to Plant Bt Corn: Farm-Level Economic Impacts of Bt Corn, 1996–2001," 2001.

11. www.organicconsumers.org/ge/ge_vs_organic.cfm

12. "New Genes and Seeds: Protestors in Europe Grow More Passionate," *New York Times* (March 14, 2000).

13. Miguel Altieri, and Peter Rosset, "Ten Reasons Why Biotechnology Will Not Ensure Food Security, Protect the Environment and Reduce Poverty in the Developing World," Food First/Institute for Food and Development (October 1999).

CHAPTER 2

1. www.organicconsumers.org/gefood/gegut071802.cfm

2. Jeffrey M. Smith, *Seeds of Deception: Exposing Industry and Government Lies About the Safety of the Genetically Engineered Foods You're Eating* (Fairfield, Iowa, Yes! Books, 2003), pp. 107–125.

3. *Maclean's* (Jan. 20, 1997) "Science: Unnatural Selection: Are Genetically Altered Foods Really Safe?" A. N. Mayeno and G. J. Gleich "Eosinophilia-Myalgia Syndrome and Tryptophan Production: A Cautionary Tale." *TIBTECH* (1994): 346–352. *Phillip Raphals Science* (November 2, 1990) "Does Medical Mystery Threaten Biotech?"

4. Ibid.

5. "Why I Cannot Remain Silent: Interview with Dr. Arpad Pusztai" *GM Free* (U.K.) (August-September 1999).

6. Quoted by Joel Bleifuss, "No Small (Genetic) Potatoes," *In These Times* (January 10, 2000).

7. "Cauliflower Mosaic Viral Promoter—A Recipe for Disaster?" *Microbial Ecology in Health and Disease* (no. 4, 1999).

8. "I Was Right, Says GM Row Scientist" (London) *Independent* (March 8, 1999); also sourced by the next footnote, *In These Times* (January 10, 2000).

9. Joel Bleifuss, "No Small (Genetic) Potatoes," *In These Times* (January 10, 2000). To see the full report by Dr. Pusztai go to www.rri.sari.ac.uk/gmo/index.html

10. Sheldon Rampton and John Stauber, *Trust Us We're Experts,* (New York, Jeremy Tarcher Putnam, 2001).

11. Julie Nordless, Steve Taylor et al., "Identification of a Brazil-Nut Allergen in Transgenic Soybeans," *The New England Journal of Medicine* (March 14, 1996).

12. Gladwell, Malcolm, "Biotech Food Products Won't Require Special Rules, FDA Decides." *Washington Post* (May 26, 1992).

13. J. Raloff, "Allergies to this Soy Would Be Nutty," *Science News*, Vol. 149 (March, 16, 1999).

14. See footnote #2 p.167.

15. Ibid. p.167.

16. Marc Kaufman, "Biotech Corn is Test Case for Industry," *Washington Post* (March 19, 2001).

17. Goldburg quote from the book *Imagine a World Without Monarch Butterflies* by Alex Jack, p. 19.

18. Rick Weiss, "Biotech Food Raises a Crop of Questions," *Washington Post* (August 15, 1999).

19. Marian Nestle, "Allergies to Transgenic Foods—Questions of Policy," *The New England Journal of Medicine* (March 14, 1996), pp. 726–27.

20. Associated Press, "U.S. Downplays European Fears over Biotech Crops," Feb. 24, 2004, www.organicconsumers.org/ge/philippine.cfm

21. Legal affidavit submitted August 12, 1998, by Dr. Mae-Wan-Ho in a UK court case on genetically engineered foods. The affidavit is posted on the Web site of the Institute of Science in Society, www.i-sis.org/

22. Shiv Chopra and others, rBST (NUTRALAC) "Gaps Analysis" Report By rBST Internal Review Team, Health Protection Branch, Health Canada (April 21, 1998). Also Frederick Bever, "Canadian Agency Questions Approval of Cow Drug by US," Rutland (Vermont) *Herald* (October 6, 1998).

23. Dr. Peter Montague, "Milk rBGH and Cancer," *Rachel's Environment and Health Weekly* #593 (April 9, 1998).

24. The *Milwaukee State Journal* (January 26, 1996).

25. "Study Casts Doubt on Genetically Modified Food," Reuters (January 28, 1999).

26. http://www.organicconsumers.org/gefood/gmdnainHumans.cfm

27. See footnote #1 in this chapter.

28. D. K. Mercer et al., "Fate of Free DNA and Transformation of the Oral Bacterium Streptococcus Gordonii DL1 by Plasmid DNA in NHuman Saliva," Applied an Environmental Microbiology 65 (1999): 6–10.

29. Julie Vorman, "Deadly E. Coli Bug May Affect Half of U.S. Cattle," Reuters (November 10, 1999).

30. Mae-Wan Ho, Terje Traavik, et al "Gene Technology & Gene Ecology of Infectious Diseases," *Microbial Ecology in Health and Disease* (Vol. 10): 33–59.

31. For an examination of USDA statistics on pesticide use by U.S. farmers growing herbicide-resistant and Bt crops in 1997–98 see the analysis by Dr. Charles Benbrook, former head of the Agriculture Committee of the National Academy of Sciences, at www.biotech-info.net.

32. L. Hardell and M. Erickson, "A Case-Control Study of non-Hodgkin's Lymphoma and Exposure to Pesticides," *Cancer* 86 (6), 1999.

33. Caroline Cox, "Glyphosate, Part I: Toxicology," *Journal of Pesticide Reform*, Fall 1995, Vol. 15 no. 3. See also "Glyphosate, Part 2: Human Exposure and Ecological Effects," *Journal of Pesticide Reform*, Vol. 14 no. 4 (Winter 1995).
34. www.organicconsumers.org/ge/monsanto_roundup_banned.cfm
35. "Ready for Roundup," *GM Free*, August/September 1999, Pagell.
36. Marc Lappe and Britt Bailey, *Against the Grain*, (Common Courage Press, 1998), p.147. A. Garcia et al., "Paternal Exposure to Pesticides and Congenital Malformations," *Scandinavian Journal of Work-Related and Environmental Health* 24 (1998): 473–80.
37. A. Garcia., "Paternal Exposure to Pesticides and Congenital Malformations," *Scandinavian Journal of Work-Related and Environmental Health* 24:473–80, 1998.
38. Marc Lappe and Britt Bailey, *Against the Grain: Biotechnology and the Corporate Takeover of Your Food* (Common Courage Press, 1998), pp. 41–47.
39. John Nichols, "The Three Mile Island of Biotech?," *The Nation*, December 30, 2002, www.organicconsumers.org/ge/121902_genetically_engineered_ biopharm.cfm
40. www.organicconsumers.org/gefood/Biopharming0702.cfm
41. See also footnote #37.
42. Andrew Pollack, "Spread of Gene-Altered Pharmaceutical Corn Spurs $3 Million Fine," *New York Times* (December 7, 2002).
43. www.organicconsumers.org/gefood/biopharm121002.cfm
44. www.biotech-info.net/health_risks.html#digestibility

CHAPTER 3

1. James Kling, "Could Transgenic Crops One Day Breed Superweeds," *Science* 274 (1994): 180–181.
2. www.guardian.co.uk/gmdebate/Story/0,2763,1055016,00.html
3. Andrew Pollack, "No Foolproof Way Is Seen to Contain Altered Genes," *New York Times* (January 21, 2004).
4. Press Release—Union of Concerned Scientists, "Genetically Engineered DNA Found in Traditional Seeds," February 23, 2004, www.organicconsumers.org /ge/contamination.cfm
5. Graeme Wilson, "Farmers told there is no escape from GM pollen," *UK Daily Mail* (January 19, 2000).
6. www.organicconsumers.org/organic/frankencrops051503.cfm
7. www.organicconsumers.org/organic/011103_0rganic.cfm7. Center for Food Safety, "Greenpeace, Center for Food Safety and Organic Farmers Sue EPA Over Gene-Altered Crops," Press Release (February 18, 1999).
8. L. Hansen and J. Obrycki, "Non-target effects of Bt corn pollen on the Monarch butterfly (Lepidoptera: Danaidae)," Iowa State University, Ames, IA. From: www.ent.iastate.edu/entoc/ncb99/prog/abs/D81.html
9. Scott Kilman, "Britain Links Biotech Crops To Lower Insect Populations," *Wall Street Journal* (October 20, 2003).
10. C. Crecchio and G. Stotzky, "Insecticidal Activity and Biodegradation of the Toxin from Bacillus Thuringiensis Subsp.Kurstaki Bound to Humic Acids from the Soil," *Soil Biology and Biochemistry* 30 (1998): 463–70.

11. D. Saxena et al., "Insecticidal Toxin in Root Exudates from Bt Corn," *Nature* 402: 480, 1999.
12. M. J. Holmes, E. R. Ingham, "The effects of genetically engineered microorganisms on soil foodwebs," *Bulletin of the Ecological Society of America*, Supplement (1994):75:97.
13. Vandana Shiva, *Biopiracy: The Plunder of Nature and Knowledge* (South End Press, 1997), 34–35.
14. Mary MacArthur, "Triple-Resistant Canola Weeds Found in Alberta," *Western Producer* (February 10, 2000).
15. *The Times-Picayune*, "Blue Revolution May Be Wave Of Future" (January 16, 2000).
16. W. M. Muir, R. D. Howard, "Possible ecological risks of transgenic organism releasewhen transgenes affect mating success: sexual selection and the Trojan gene hypothesis," *PNAS* 96 (1999):13853–56.
17. Associated Press, "New Zealand firm promises to stop breeding 'Frankenfish' " (February 27, 2000).
18. Keith Schneider, "Go Ahead Likely on Crop Tinkering, But Some Are Wary," The *New York Times* (May 25, 1994).
19. www.organicconsumers.org/ge/monsanto121503.cfm
20. Ibid.
21. www.organicconsumers.org/toxic/riddleonhogs.cfm

CHAPTER 4

1. Michael Fox, *Eating with Conscience: The Bioethics of Food* (NewSage Press, 1997), 76.
2. Research Advancement Foundation International, "AgBiotech's Five Jumbo Gene Giants," January 7, 2000, www.rafi.org.
3. Martin Teitel and Kimberly Wilson, *Genetically Engineered Food: Changing the Nature of Nature* (Park Street Press, 1999), 16.
4. Richard A. Shanks and Joseph Mendelson, "Crops or Courts: Farmers Bear Risks Associated with Genetically Altered Seed Crops," *Texas Lawyer* (July 1, 2002).
5. Sue Branford, "Soy Resistant," The Guardian (London), April 17, 2002. http://www.organicconsumers.org/gefood/brazilsoya042302.cfm
6. Peter Kendall, "Engineered Crops Face Barren Season, Farmers Fear Controversy Over Genetically Altered Seed May Make Harvest Unmarketable," *Chicago Tribune* (January 24, 2000).
7. Andrew Pollack, "No Foolproof Way is Found to Contain Altered Genes," *New York Times* (Jan. 21, 2004).
8. General Accounting Office, "Biotechnology—Information on Prices of Genetically Modified Seeds in the United States and Argentina," Washington, D.C., January 2000.
9. Kevin Gray, "Monsanto Halts Sales of Soybean Sales in Argentina Because of Illicit Cultivation," Associated Press (Jan. 19, 2004).
10. Kristen Philipkoski, "Food Biotech Is Risky Business," *Wired News* (Dec 01, 2003).
11. J. L. Fox, 1997. "Farmers Say Monsanto's Engineered Cotton Drops Bolls." *Nature Biotechnology*, 15: 1233.

12. Michael Hansen, "Genetic Engineering Is Not An Extension of Conventional Plant Breeding," Consumer Policy Institute (January 27, 2000). Submitted to the Food and Drug Administration.
13. www.organicconsumers.org/ge/monsanto121503.cfm
14. Mike Lee, "Seeds of Worry on Roundup," *Sacramento Bee* (Nov. 12, 2003).
15. Peter Montague, "Sustainability and Ag Biotech," *Rachel's Environment & Health Weekly*, #686 (February 10, 2000).
16. www.organicconsumers.org/newsletter/biod38.cfm
17. www.greenpeaceusa.org/media/press_releases/2003/04162003.htm
18. Ibid.
19. Willard Cochrane, "A Food and Agricultural Policy for the 21st Century," *Institute for Agriculture and Trade Policy* (February 2000).
20. Associated Press, "Too Few Farmers Left to Count, Agency Says" (October 10, 1993).
21. Nikki Tait, "Farmers Ponder Seed Options: Larger U.S. Farms Are Tending to Plant GM Crops While Smaller Concerns Are Looking for a Non-GM Premium," *The Financial Times* (March 7, 2000).
22. Brewster Kneen, *Farmageddon: Food and the Culture of Biotechnology* (New Society Publishers, 1999).
23. Associated Press, "There Are as Many People Overweight in World as Underfed" (March 5, 2000).
24. Vandana Shiva, *Biopiracy: The Plunder of Nature and Knowledge* (South End Press, 1997).
25. Andrew Kimbrell, *"Biocolonization," The Case Against the Global Economy*, (Sierra Club Books, 1996), 133.
25. Vandana Shiva, *Biopiracy*, 55.

CHAPTER 5

1. Center for Food Safety, lawsuit filed May 27, 1998. Federal Court, Washington, DC.
2. Linda Bren, "Genetic Engineering: The Future of Foods?" *FDA Consumer Magazine* (November/December 2003).
3. Statement of Rebecca Goldburg, Environmental Defense Fund, at the FDA Public Hearing on Genetically Engineered Foods. November 30, 1999, Washington, D.C.
4. Ben Lilliston, "Aiding and Abetting—U.S. Regulatory System Turns Blind Eye Toward Genetically Engineered Foods," *Multinational Monitor* (January/February 2000).
5. Ibid.
6. Comments from Dr. Linda Kahl, FDA compliance officer, to Dr. James Maryanski, FDA Biotechnology Coordinator, about the federal register document "Statement of Policy: Foods from Genetically Modified Plants." Dated January 8, 1992. Can be viewed at: www.biointegrity.org
7. Comments from Dr. Louis J. Pribyl re: the "Biotechnology Draft Document, 2/27/92." Dated March 6, 1992. Can be viewed at: www.biointegrity.org.

8. Associated Press, "Better Study Is Urged Of Biotech Crops' Effects" (February 18, 2000).

9. Center for Food Safety, lawsuit filed February 18, 1999, against U.S. Environmental Protection Agency. Can be viewed at: www.centerforfoodsafety.org/li/BT2ndam.html.

10. Rebecca Goldburg, Environmental Defense Fund. Testimony before the U.S. House of Representatives Committee on Science's Subcommittee on Basic Research (October 1999).

11. Center for Science in the Public Interest, Press Release, September 10, 2003. http://cspinet.org/new/200309101.html

12. Ben Lilliston, "Aiding and Abetting—U.S. Regulatory System Turns Blind Eye Toward Genetically Engineered Foods," *Multinational Monitor* (January/February 2000).

13. Rick Weiss, "Next Food Fight Brewing Over Listing Genes on Labels." *Washington Post* (August 15, 1999).

14. Center for Food Safety Press Release, November 12, 2003. www.centerforfood-safety.org/BiopharmRelease.pdf

15. Friends of the Earth, questions and answers on biopharming. www.foe.org/bio-pharm/qanda.html#reg

16. Union of Concerned Scientists, Web feature—Environmental Effects of Genetically Modified Food Crops Recent Experiences. www.ucsusa.org/food_and_environ-ment/biotechnology/page.cfm?pageID=1219

17. Food and Drug Administration, "Statement of Policy: Foods Derived From New Plant Varieties," *Federal Register*, Vol. 57. No. 104 (May 29, 1992), 229991.

18. Coca-Cola, November 9, 1999, letter from Kathy Daly, consumer affairs specialist to Debbie Ortman.

CHAPTER 6

1. Union of Concerned Scientists. Updated November 1999. Web site: www.uscusa.org.

2. Claire Robinson, "GM Animal Feed: No regulation, no segregation; no choice," *GM-FREE*, Vol. 1 No. 4 (November/December 1999), 4.

3. Mothers for Natural Law. Much of this information can be found at the Mothers for Natural Law Web site: www.safefood.org.

4. Joanna Blythman, *How To Avoid GM Foods* (Fourth Estate, London. 1999), 58.

5. Ibid, 61.

6. Ibid, 68-71.

7. *Consumer Reports* (September 1999).

8. Top 1000 U.S. Corporations, *Fortune Magazine* (April 14, 2003).

9. Greenpeace report, *FDA Approved: Genetically Engineered Soy and Corn in Baby Food and Nutritional Supplements* (June 10, 1999).

10. Scott Kilman, "USA: Monsanto's Biotech Spud Is Being Pulled from the Fryer at Fast-Food Chain," *Wall Street Journal* (April 28, 2000).

11. "McCain blows cool on GM potatoes," *Farmer's Weekly* (December 3, 1999).

CHAPTER 7

1. Brett Chase, "Whole Foods, Wild Oats Chains to Ban Gene-Altered Ingredients," Bloomberg News Service (December 30, 1999).
2. Lucette Lagnado, "Gerber Baby Food, Grilled by Greenpeace, Plans Swift Overhaul," *Wall Street Journal* (July 30, 1999).
3. Scott Kilman, "USA: Monsanto's Biotech Spud Is Being Pulled from the Fryer at Fast-Food Chain, " *Wall Street Journal* (April 28, 2000).
4. Scott Kilman, "Biotech Scare Sweeps Europe, and Companies Wonder If U.S. Is Next," *Wall Street Journal* (October 7, 1999).
5. Ibid.
6. "Seagram Co. Tells Farmers It Won't Buy Genetically Modified Corn," *Toronto Star* (February 9, 2000).
7. Soyatech. "ADM opens organic soy processing facility in North Dakota." December 9, 2003. www.soyatech.com/bluebook/news/viewarticle.ldml?a=20031209-6)
8. Alex Jack, *Imagine a World Without Monarch Butterflies* (One Peaceful World Press 2000).
9. Greenpeace Press Release. December 20, 1999. "U.K. Supermarkets Move Out of GM-fed Animal Products. U.K.'s largest retailer, Tesco, pulling out in 2000."
10. Andrew Pollack, "Maker Warns of Scarcity of Hormone for Dairy Cows." The *New York Times* (January 27, 2004).
11. Martin Teitel, and Kimberly Wilson. *Genetically Engineered Food: Changing the Nature of Nature* (Park Street Press, 1999), 35.
12. E-mail from Jennifer K. DeClue, R.D., Nutrition Specialist, Office of Consumer Affairs, Purina (January 5, 2000).

CHAPTER 8

1. John Fetto, "Home on the Organic Range," *American Demographics* (August 1999).
2. Catherine Greene, and Carolyn Dimitri. "Amber Waves," USDA's Economic Research Service, February 2003, www.ers.usda.gov/amberwaves/feb03/findings/organicagriculture.htm.
3. The World of Organic Agriculture 2004—Statistics and Future Prospects, February 2004.
4. Jens-Otto Anderson, "Farming, Plant Nutrition and Food Quality," Presentation to the Soil Association (January 3, 2000). Also, BBC News, "Organic Food 'Proven' Healthier" (January 3, 2000).
5. Cheryl Long, "Open Letter to the USDA," *Organic Gardening Magazine* (November/December 1999).
6. John Spitler, "New Evidence Organic Crops may be Healthier." *Farm Progress* (March 19, 2003).
7. American Chemical Society. "Research at Great Lakes Meeting Shows More Vitamin C in Organic Oranges Than Conventional Organges," June 2, 2002, www.sciencedaily.com/releases/2002/06/020603071017.htm
8. "Eating Organic Food May Help Reduce Your Risk of Heart Attacks, Strokes and Cancer." *New Scientist* (March 14, 2002). www.newscientist.com/news/news.jsp?id=ns99992033

9. Allison Byrum, "Organically Grown Foods Higher In Cancer-fighting Chemicals Than Conventionally Grown Foods," *Eurekalert* (March 3, 2003).
10. Cheryl Long, "Open Letter to the USDA," *Organic Gardening Magazine* (November/December 1999).
11. Andrew Pollack, "No Foolproof Way Is Seen to Contain Altered Genes," *New York Times* (January 21, 2004).
12. Donal Kinney, "Southwest Cooperative Grocers Association Meets in Albuquerque," Co-op Connection, Albuquerque, NM.
13. Sustainable Agriculture Research and Education (SARE) Program, January 5, 2000, Press Release, "New Directory Links Farmers, Consumers in Food Partnerships."
14. Kirk Johnson, "Bringing in the Harvest, Without a Farm in Sight." *New York Times* (October 27, 2003).
15. Oliver Ludwig, "Farmers Markets Sprout Up Across America," Reuters (September 1999).
16. Lucette Lagnado, "U.S. Restaurants Try To End Genetically Modified Food," *The Wall Street Journal* (March 9, 2000).

ACKNOWLEDGMENTS

MANY INDIVIDUALS and organizations helped in the writing of this book. The list is too long to name everyone. But here are a few people whose assistance was greatly appreciated: Gabriela Flora, Marnie Glickman, Michael Hansen, Simon Harris, Andy Kimbrell, Judy Linman, Charles Margulis, Loranda McLeet, Joe Mendelson, Ana Micka, Sarah Newport, Karen Smith, John Stauber, and Rose Welch.

We'd like to extend a special thank-you to our editor, Matthew Lore, for his enthusiasm and commitment to this book.